Life201
SEXUAL HEALTH

HARNESS YOUR SEXUAL ENERGY, LIVE YOUR BEST LIFE

Adiel Gorel with
seven health experts

IDEAL LIFE PRESS
SAN RAFAEL, CALIFORNIA

Ideal Life Press
165 North Redwood Drive, Ste #150
San Rafael, CA 94903
ideallifepress.com
info@ideallifepress.com
life201.com

This book is for educational purposes only. It is not intended as a substitute for medical or financial advice. Please consult a qualified health care professional for individual health and medical advice, and please consult a qualified financial professional for financial advice. Neither Ideal Life Press nor any author shall have any responsibility for any adverse effects arising directly or indirectly as a result of the information provided in this book.

This book contains the ideas and opinions of its authors. The strategies outlined in this book may not be suitable for every individual and are not guaranteed or warranted to produce any particular results. No warranty is made with respect to the accuracy or completeness of the information contained herein, and the authors, the publisher (Ideal Life Press), Life201, Inc., Allusa Investments, Inc., and International Capital Group (ICG) specifically disclaim any responsibility for any liability, loss or risk, personal or otherwise, which is incurred as a consequence, directly or indirectly, of the use and application of any of the contents of this book.

Throughout this book, trademark names are used. Rather than put a trademark symbol after every occurrence of a trademark name, we use names in an editorial fashion only, and to the benefit of the trademark owner, with no intention of infringement of the trademark.

Life 201 SEXUAL HEALTH: Harness your sexual energy,
live your best life / Adiel Gorel. — 1st edition.
ISBN 979-8-9907840-0-0 softcover edition
Library of Congress Control Number 2023918485

ACKNOWLEDGMENTS

I am very fulfilled by creating this guide for a richer and fuller life, with the expert partners who generously shared their knowledge in the chapters of this book.

Naturally, it took a village to accomplish this task.

Thanks to the incredible experts who joined me in creating this useful resource on sexual wellness for everyone:

Thanks to Dr. Felice Gersh for teaching us about hormones, and how overall health as well as sexual health can be improved.

Thanks to Navin Ramachandran for lifting the veil on online dating, one of the biggest relationship creators nowadays.

Thanks to Dr. Vicki Matthews for teaching us how to use the Five Elements model for better relationships.

Thanks to Margot Anand who taught us to use sexual energies to enhance our spiritual growth, among many other benefits.

Thanks to Ulises Calatayud for teaching us about the practical aspects of Tantra, with benefits to health and happiness, with tangible examples.

Thanks to Dr. Kelly Casperson for dispelling many outdated sexual myths and showing us that sex can be fulfilling for everyone, at any age.

Thanks to Dr. Siyamak Saleh for busting myths our kids are bombarded with on social media, and helping people get sane ideas about sexuality and sex.

Thanks to Kim Anami, who does not have a chapter in this book, but my interview with her is part of the summit. Kim talks about improved sexual function and health.

Many thanks to the team at my company, in the U.S. and abroad, for their constant support of our investors and for making the operation run smoothly, enabling me to have the time to create this book as well as other helpful content. Special thanks to Ciarra Herrell, Kristi Sessi, Lauralee Butler Reinke, and Carmit Sharaby.

Thanks to the talented and amazing team at Heightener, in particular Camper Bull, Canon Wing, Lorraine Evans, and Ilya Farahmand. The Heightener team is the backbone of the summit, our podcast, and our outreach to the outside world. They are tireless and very effective.

Thanks to Chad Lefevre, who creates the structure around our podcast interviews, reaches out to the speakers, and makes the podcasts happen, while also being present during the interviews. Chad makes the podcast and the summit feel comfortable, letting each speaker worry only about speaking and nothing else.

Thanks to Erin Saxton for reaching out to many of our interviewees and inviting them to join our ever-growing universe of top experts with highly useful information. Erin's gravitas, coupled with her gregarious demeanor, helps me connect with many fascinating interviewees.

Thanks to Jerry Adams, who was a driving force behind the public television show Life 201, and has since been key to the development of our books, including this book about the Life 201 Sexual Wellness Summit. Jerry leaves no stone unturned, and has a keen eye on deadlines, production, and performance.

Thanks to Paul Pavlovich for the design of the book, making some complex medical information readable and accessible.

Thanks to Ruth Schwartz of Wonderlady Books for her editing and publishing expertise.

And last but not least, special thanks to my children, Daphne and Daniel. You are a constant source of inspiration. I keep learning from you, and I appreciate that you also tolerate your often-busy dad. I love you!

CONTENTS

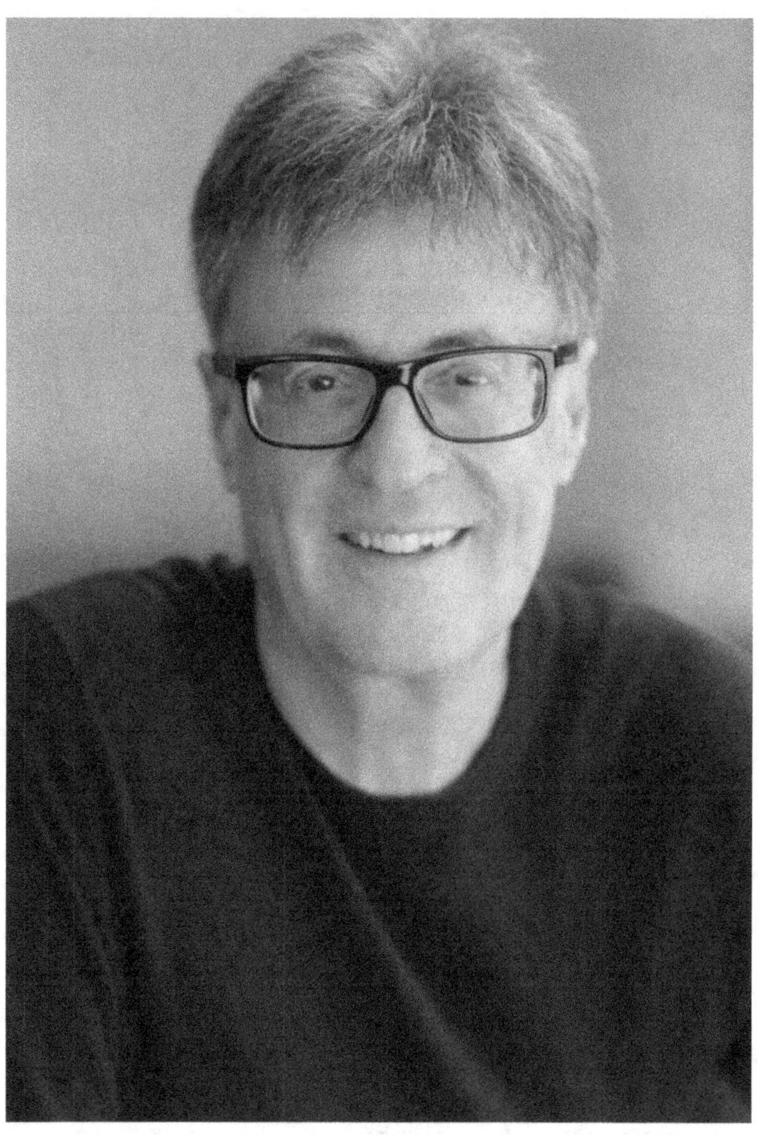

Adiel Gorel

CHAPTER 1

INTRODUCTION

By Adiel Gorel

Sexuality is looked upon differently in various cultures throughout the world. Some consider any mention of sexual energy or overall sexuality taboo. There are body and spiritual work modalities which attempt to harness the power of our sexuality to heal and perhaps reach higher levels of consciousness. In my world travels, I have seen the disparity between different cultures' attitudes and beliefs about sex and sexuality.

It cannot be denied that sexual energy is very powerful. It is part of human physiology and psychology. Sexual energy affects our behavior, and our relationships, and is the energy that leads to procreation.

It is clear that sexual energy generates heat and power. Some practitioners of Tantra claim that sexual energy, properly channeled, is responsible for what we call "charisma."

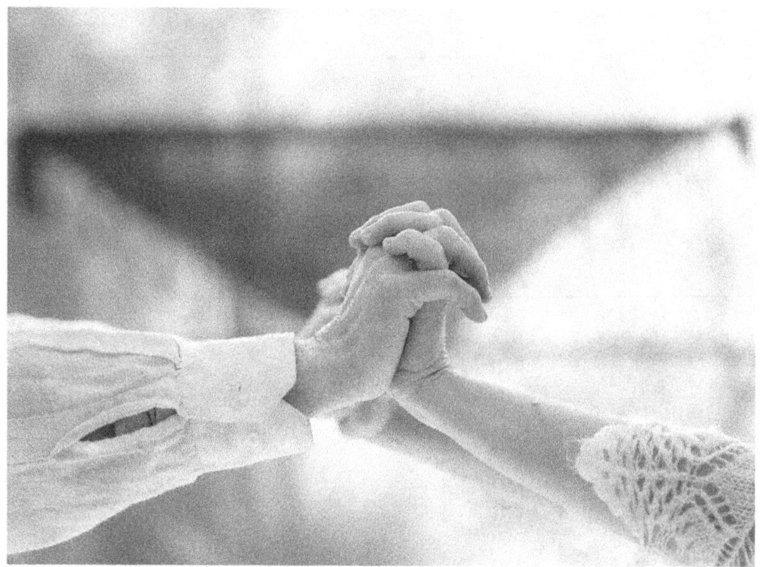

As part of being a constant seeker of health and wellness, I explored the potential of Tantra myself. I took workshops with Mantak Chia, after reading his book *Taoists Secrets of Love: Cultivating Male Sexual Energy*. In the workshops, he explored the cultivation of both male and female sexual energy. I have retained some of the teachings to this day and thought the workshops were useful for a healthy life in general as well.

I also took workshops from Charles Muir, after reading his book *Tantra, the Art of Conscious Loving*. His workshops resonated with the Mantak Chia materials and added Charles' own layers. Those too were useful and interesting.

Much of humanity looks at sexuality and sexual energy as just another facet of our bodily functions, to be discussed with discretion.

Sexual dysfunction in both males and females is usually treated via drugs and/or surgery, similar to other bodily issues, especially in the West. Due to the more discreet nature of sexual issues, both positive and negative, some people may be harboring misconceptions about whether they are "okay" sexually. That is especially true in the later stages of life.

The private nature of sexuality, which hampers many people from seeking help if they need it, can create shame, feeling "broken" and inadequate, and at a loss for help. Some people simply shut down the sexual side of their life, regarding it as a source of guilt and potential failure.

Normal changes in later life can create anxiety and frustration, especially when not dealt with in an open and productive way. We hope to show that these feelings are not necessarily called for and that almost everyone can enjoy a fulfilling sex life, even if it doesn't conform to one narrow definition of what "sex" is.

On our Life201 Podcast *The Adiel Gorel Show*, we interview experts in various aspects of wellness, fitness, and longevity.

We were fortunate to have several inspiring experts on the subject of sexual wellness. That motivated us to put forth our Sexual Wellness Summit. Each of the experts contributed a chapter to this book, which we hope will prove to be a useful reference for all of us.

The information content is not only for heterosexual sex, but for anybody who is interested in improving their sexual experience, and using sexual energy to elevate health, wellness—and perhaps even spirituality—regardless of their gender identity, love partner, or orientation.

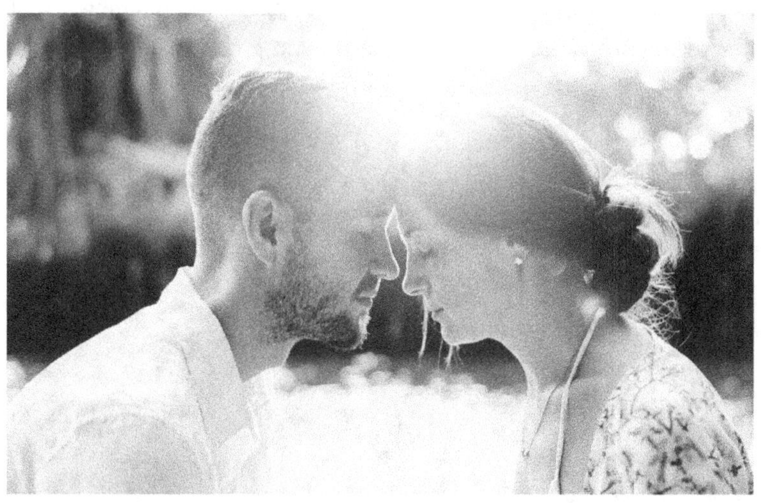

The various experts participating in the summit span a range of areas within the "Sexual Wellness" universe.

Dr. Felice Gersh is an expert on female and male issues, hormone levels, and what comprises sexual wellness. She will enlighten us as to appropriate levels of both estrogen and testosterone in both males and females and highlight health-promoting advice.

Navin Ramachandran takes us into the online dating world, having been a high-level executive in the Match Group of dating websites.

Dr. Vicki Matthews talks about the five elements of nature and how we each have one or more of these elements as a dominant feature. She will discuss how, in a relationship, it is beneficial to understand your elements—as well as your partner's—to achieve greater relationship harmony.

Margot Anand, the author of *The Art of Sexual Ecstasy*, as well as many other books on Tantra, is a renowned Tantra teacher, who explores Tantra for spiritual growth, among many other benefits.

Ulises Calatayud is a tantric master who, in fact, had initially studied with Margo Anand. He talks about harnessing sexual energy for health and spiritual development, with some tangible examples.

Dr. Kelly Casperson dispels many myths about what "sex" is supposed to be and shows us how everyone can and should have a fulfilling sexual life, regardless of the stage of life they are in.

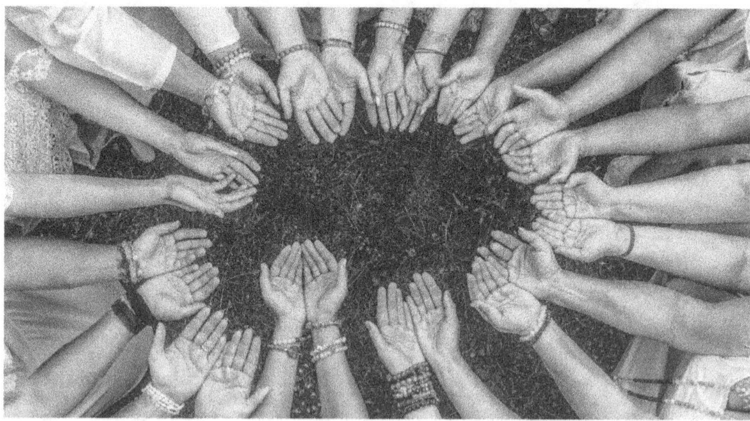

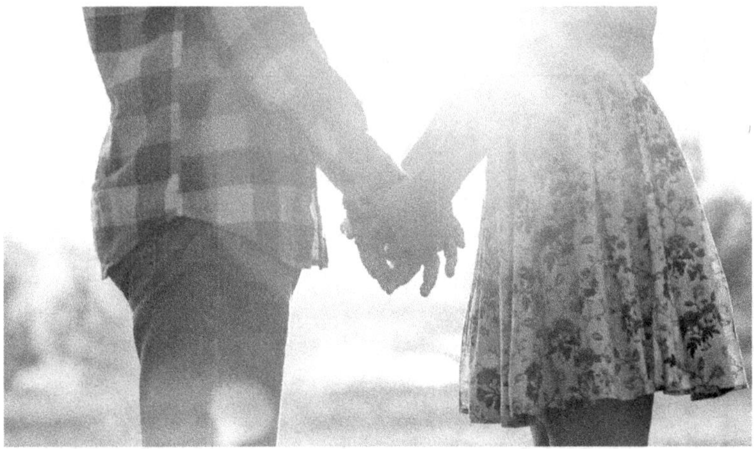

Dr. Siyamak Saleh debunks many myths relating to human sexuality, including many widespread common myths that abound in many cultures.

Kim Anami does not have a chapter in this book but has been interviewed. In her interview, she covers sexual function improvement and lays the path to a fulfilling sexual life.

All these interviews were interesting and illuminating, covering various facets of an area of life that usually stays under the covers (pun intended) for much of the world.

We are grateful to these busy experts for sharing their experiences and knowledge with us on the podcast, and in the chapters they contributed to the book. Our team extends deep gratitude to the experts who contributed to us: the readers, viewers, and listeners. The condensed version of one chapter per expert also is in harmony with how busy we all are these days, and how digesting an expert's knowledge is easier when it is contained in a single chapter.

We hope you have enjoyed the Sexual Wellness Summit, and that you will enjoy this book as well.

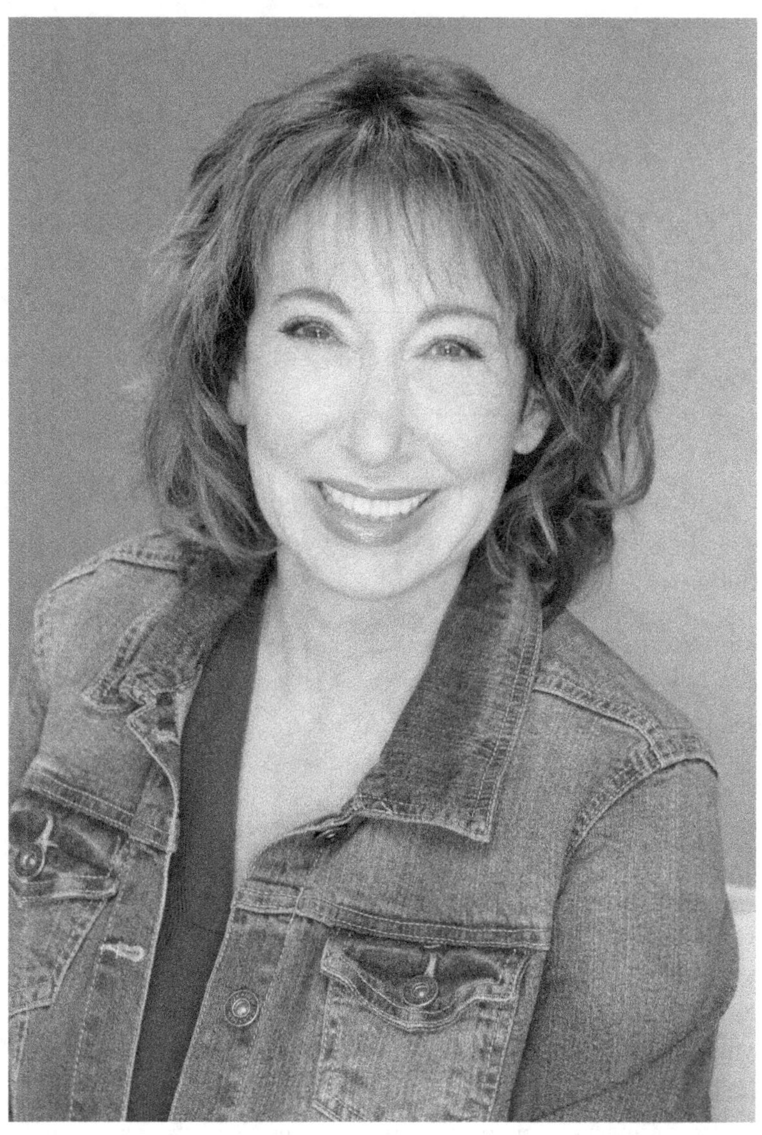

Dr. Felice Gersh

CHAPTER 2

LIFE'S PRIMARY DIRECTIVE: They tell you in medical school, "Half of what you learn in medical school is wrong, but you don't know which half that was." It is a little scary to think that we could be receiving medical treatment that isn't as sound as we need it to be. When the prime directive of life is to create new life, every system in the body is actually geared towards procreation. Humans are the only species that try to control and limit this process. What if the meds, contraceptives, and other products we use are fundamentally incompatible with our well-being? What if part of what we learned in medical school that was wrong is fundamental to our prime directive in life?

SEXUAL HEALTH IS A PREDICTOR OF OVERALL QUALITY OF LIFE

By Dr. Felice Gersh

Think of how the urge to have sex drives all animals. The dog of a friend of mine wasn't spayed. When in heat, that dog wanted to hump everything in sight, even a convenient human leg if there was no actual dog available. Friends would bring along their male dogs— one of those dogs even ran away squealing when he couldn't keep up. She was insatiable. However, in a couple of weeks, it was all over, and my friend's dog was back to her usual self.

We humans don't function like that. We see sex as more than just the reproductive instinct. It is also about relationships, bonding, and intimacy. We are among the few species that engage in recreational sex, which makes sexual function even more central to our well-being.

Sexual desire and function are important and very complex

As an OB-GYN who has delivered thousands of babies in my career, I know that the prime directive of life is the creation of new life. This requires having sex, so sexuality is a key driver of both behavior and health. Hormones regulate desire and sexual function. There are many other contributors, but our hormones are foundational.

However, unlike animals, we humans spend a lot of our lives trying to prevent reproduction. We use hormonal interventions to do this, which then interferes with the natural sex drive. Hormone-based contraceptives have, of course, been a major instrument for liberation, but they are also seen to inhibit optimal sexual desire and function. They are major endocrine disruptors that interfere with ovarian functioning and actually disturb the hormonal environment and balance.

Sexual function and the things that disrupt it

When the body finds that the normal production of hormones is impeded, it behaves differently, it reacts differently to stimuli. Over the years, researchers have found that being on the pill can have all kinds of unforeseen fallouts for sexual health.

Pheromones are chemical messengers that living creatures excrete to communicate with each other. A study found that the pill can disrupt pheromone production, which contributes significantly to sexual and romantic attraction.[1] In humans, this function is subtle but important. Not only does the pill seem to inhibit pheromone production, it also alters how female receptors respond to male pheromones. According to the study, a woman could literally choose one partner over another simply because she is on the pill!

Ovulation, which is blocked by the pill, also impacts subconscious male attraction. In another study, men demonstrated a marked preference for the ovulating woman.[2] This 2011 study examined the impact of ovulation on male behavior and found that subtle signs of women's fertility influenced the mating cognition and behavior of males.

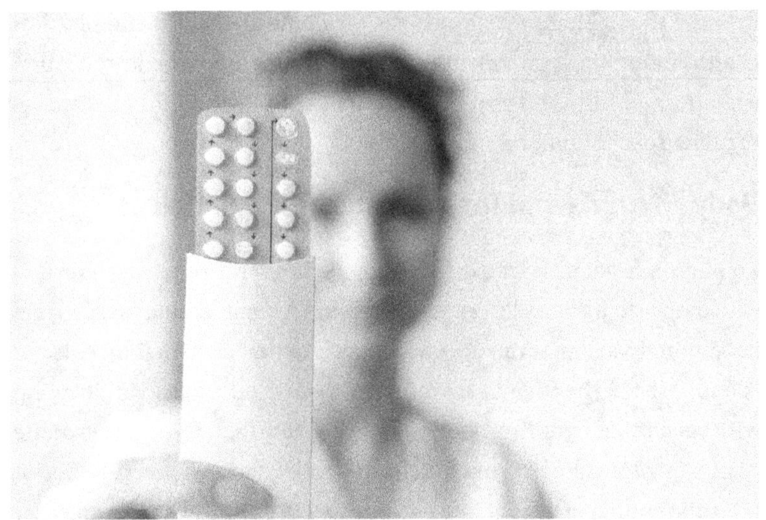

Yet another study examined the effects of the ovulatory cycle on tip earnings by lap dancers. This study found that women near the most fertile point of their menstrual cycle seemed to be more attractive to men. The study noted that men were found to tip women significantly more when they were ovulating than at other times in their cycle. By contrast, women on the pill saw no such increase in earnings. Clearly, there were subtle cues that men were picking up on, which made women more attractive to them at some times than at other times.

With so many women taking the pill for most of their reproductive lives —at times starting as early as 13 or 14 years of age—many are *never* able to experience their natural sex drive and attraction. Unfortunately, this is something that we are not talking about enough.

Studies over the years have shown us that the pill tends to impact mood and can contribute to mental illness. For instance, estrogen and progesterone are seen to influence neurochemistry, brain function, and the activity of certain neurotransmitters. There is also evidence to suggest that the hormone progesterone can impact mood. While it is true that newer types of contraceptive pills have a weaker link to mood problems, these cannot be discounted entirely. There is still sound evidence to suggest that hormonal contraception can precipitate or perpetuate depression in some patients.

Because the pill has negative effects on women's mental and physical health, I am a big proponent of the barrier method of contraception whenever feasible and appropriate because of the way that hormones regulate sexual function.

Body rhythms and the rhythms of the universe

To maintain healthy sexual function, we probably ought to interfere with nature to the smallest extent possible. Over millennia, the ancients have noted various impacts on sexual function. For instance, there is support for the idea that women's menstrual cycles will sync up with each other over time and frequently even align to the cycle of the dominant woman of a group, such as in college-age women in a dorm. Over the course of a few months, they would all start cycling together and have their periods at the same time. There is also a connection to universal rhythms, such as the lunar cycle.

We also see how women's cycles often correspond to lunar cycles— it is no coincidence that the lunar cycle is 28 days and that most women's cycles are also 28 days. Women typically experience elevated testosterone levels around ovulation, which increases sex drive. We also observe how the female cycle can impact testosterone production in men. All of this probably explains why the full moon is tied so closely

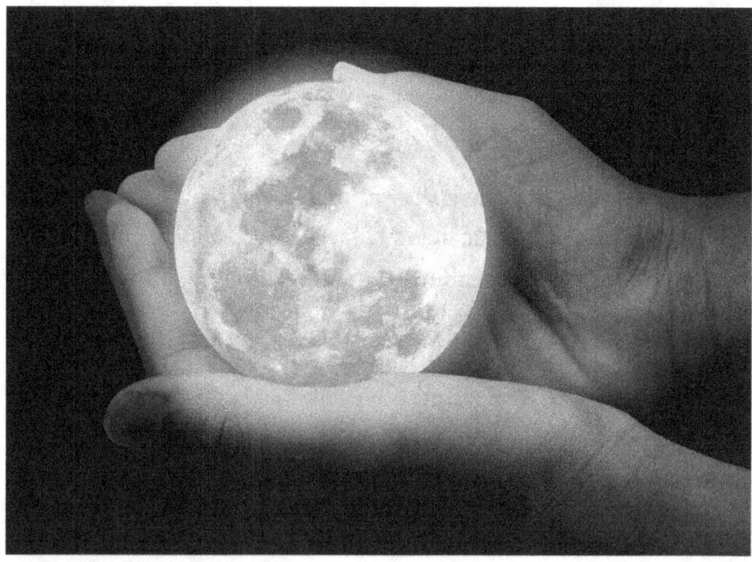

to romance in so many cultures. If people are having more sex on full moon nights, there is a reason for this!

Day and night, the seasons, the waxing and waning of the moon have more of an impact on our sexual health than we probably realize. The kind of lives we live, with climate-controlled interiors, artificial light, and blue-lit screens constantly blinking up at us, are far removed from what nature intended. We no longer permit our sexual selves to flow with these natural biorhythms. Perhaps the cycles of the sun and the moon no longer impact us in the way that they should.

Take the example of zoos and the way they have evolved over time. When they used to have small cramped cages for animal pairs, they found that the animals were not mating as they would in the wild. This likely was because the animals were unable to comprehend day and night or the passage of seasons fully. This is probably one of the reasons they switched to zoos with more natural environments and open spaces to encourage animals to mate and reproduce.

Contact and connection with the natural world are important elements of human sexual health. Unfortunately, we've taken humans out of their natural environment and put them into little cubicles where they rarely see the light of day—literally. Earlier, it was factories with no sunlight. Now it's made even worse by the artificial light of the screens we surround ourselves with. We are completely cut off from our natural environment, and our circadian rhythms are messed up.

I tell my patients, whenever possible, to go out and watch the sunset. The colors of the sunset—the oranges, the yellows, and the red tones—actually lower cortisol. The desire to lower cortisol and raise the production of melatonin is instilled in the body. We know how melatonin promotes sleep. Now we also know that the ovaries have receptors for melatonin. This is why getting proper sleep is connected to healthier eggs, better fertility, and a better sex life. So, going out and watching the sunrise and the sunset and then having a romantic evening with candlelight (not artificial light) can actually improve your sex drive. Women with fertility problems can improve their ability to ovulate and have better-quality eggs by adopting this practice.

We know that people are happier and calmer out in nature with the trees, sky, and clouds. Nature improves mood, and there is an obvious relationship between mood and sexuality. Depressed people are not highly sexual people. The epidemic of people on antidepressants like SSRIs further reduces libido and sexual function.

Is it any wonder that infertility is now at a never heard of before high, with male testosterone levels and sperm counts plummeting? It's all linked together. When we see how procreation is the prime directive of life, every other aspect of health tends to link back to this.

Sex is health-giving, not just life-giving

As I always say, procreation is the prime directive of life, and as such, the human body is geared toward keeping itself in optimal sexual health. Having sex lowers a man's risk of heart attacks, and regular sexual function lowers his risk of prostate cancer. Having sex is healthy so long as you practice safe sex and protect against STIs. It drives up your heartbeat and regulates hormones directly involved in sexual response, such as oxytocin. This has a calming effect by inducing happy and peaceful emotions and increasing people's bonds with each other.

Essentially, two people have great sex, look at each other and love each other, and fall asleep in each other's arms. None of this happens if you don't actually have sex and orgasms. Our society makes it harder and harder for people to have optimal sexual lives, and that is heartbreaking.

Men and testosterone

As our lifestyles and habits tend to interrupt the production of female hormones, the same is true for male hormone production, such as testosterone. Testosterone isn't just important for the libido, it regulates many other functions in the body. The brain has receptors that trigger peptides and other neurotransmitters linked to the sex drive. In addition, testosterone is also important because it converts into estradiol in the vascular system, like in arteries.

This connects to erectile dysfunction, which is a problem that comes with aging and sometimes shows up even in younger men. For erections to occur, not only does a man need to have a significant amount of testosterone but he also needs to have low levels of inflammation. This allows for proper conversion of testosterone into estradiol. This, in turn, facilitates the production of the enzyme endothelial nitric oxide synthase to make nitric oxide, which then allows vasodilation. This is when the arteries open up and engorge the penis to create an erection.

Several constituents come together to create healthy erectile function: an anti-inflammatory lifestyle, proper nutrients to make nitric oxide, and good vascular health. Pumping testosterone isn't enough. You need vitamin C and other critical micronutrients as well. You need to look at the global health of the male and the status of his vascular system: whether he has rigid heart arteries, inflammation, whether he is nutrient deficient, and whether he is getting enough nitric oxide (which is a gas antioxidant signaling agent).

Let's talk about Viagra.® How does that even work? It works by actually increasing nitric oxide, and rather than popping pills, it makes sense to do this naturally as much as possible.

So, holistic health is important, and sexual health is at the center of it all. Testosterone is the key ingredient for men. For instance, when men are put on testosterone blockers to treat prostate cancer, they sort of wilt away. Not only do they lose their sex drive, but they lose their vitality and vigor, which also impacts the brain. The brain, which is the director of the whole body, is where desire is born. That is why proper brain function, which involves testosterone converting into estradiol as well as testosterone receptors, is important. That is why proper sleep and fitness are vital.

Testosterone levels, sex drive, and fertility peak in a man's 20s and wanes as he ages. Many men will have significantly low testosterone once they are over 50 years of age. By age 60, the average man's testosterone level has dropped by 60%. However, exercise, avoiding toxins and endocrine disruptors in the environment, and eating a healthy diet can be extremely beneficial and go a long way toward restoring testosterone levels. This can mean better sexual health and fertility, better testicular function and sperm quality, and, of course, better sex!

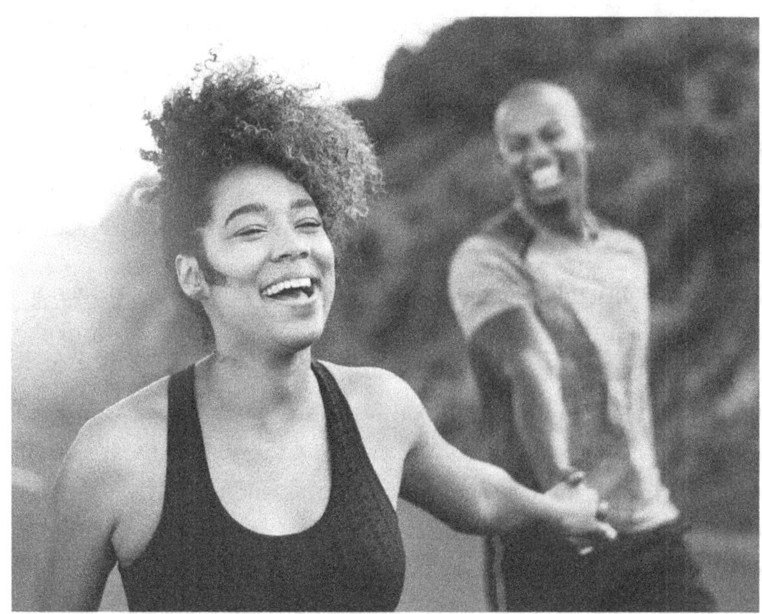

Defining one's destiny

One could argue that genetics play a big role in health and wellness. While genetic tendencies do determine a lot, there is still much that we can do to change that destiny, to define a destiny that is measurably better. We can make better choices and maintain good sexual health and fertility, which has a strong correlation with overall health. Understanding the interconnectedness of our insides is key.

I have seen men in their 60s with testosterone levels of much younger men. They produce their own testosterone naturally, maintain good vascular and cognitive health, and enjoy better moods. They have great muscle tone, which is so important for so many different functions in the body. A healthy musculoskeletal system and strong muscles are signaling agents for brain health, glucose regulation, burning sugar, and so on. Muscle mass is important to transform food into energy and prevent it from being stored as fat.

For a lot of people, aging means a big belly, low energy levels, feeling low, a flagging sex drive, and erectile dysfunction. It doesn't have to be that way. In my experience, men in their 60s can have great muscles, high energy levels, and elevated mood. Simply by having a healthy lifestyle with regular exercise, eating the right foods, and maintaining the body, you can be 100 and run a marathon! You don't have to let age be your destiny, you can change it. While you may not have the same libido as in your 20s, you can still define your destiny rather than surrender to it.

Helping the body access sufficient nitric oxide is one of the ways to do this. We get this molecule from the food we eat, particularly food high in nitrates such as green leafy veggies, beets, and so on. The right stomach acids and mouth and gut microbiome help us create nitric oxide. It is also produced by the immune system where it is transformed into a toxin to help fight invading pathogens.

Not only is it important to eat the right foods, but it is also important to maintain good digestive health in other ways. Proton-pump inhibitors or PPI drugs that dilute stomach acids could make the stomach environment suboptimal. Use of some toothpastes or mouthwashes in general similarly disturbs the oral microbiome by destroying bacteria—the good along with the bad—and are best avoided. I recommend a probiotic toothpaste by a company called Designs for Health to avoid this disturbance in the oral microbiome.

Sexual health and wellness during the later years

If a man is getting erections, this is not necessarily a sign of good vascular health. For instance, someone using Viagra could be achieving this, but it is a little like tricking the body. If there is inflammation in the body, that is going to cause all sorts of problems such as leaky gut, something we can call leaky arteries, edema, and so on. I often recommend patients undergo a microalbumin test to figure out the issue in such cases. So, testosterone shots are not going to do it. We need to go a lot deeper into the nutrient status of the man and his overall global health.

While male sexual health largely hinges on erectile function, it is more complicated and subtler for women. Arousal in men tends to be faster and more linear, but with women, it can be somewhat circular and can take time. For women, the hormones estrogen and testosterone have to work properly in conjunction for optimal sexual health. Men also need estrogen and women also need testosterone, which is important for the engorgement and sensation in the clitoris.

Though women *have* been seen to respond positively to topical testosterone gels/creams or even low doses of Viagra, the female system is definitely more complicated. There is also the fact that while male arousal is simple and direct, female arousal will often take a more persuasive route. She may need to be made to feel safe and loved and may need that bit of wooing and romance for her to get into the mood. In other words, men are somewhat less discriminating.

Female sexuality is further complicated by the way it progresses or rather transitions into menopause. The menopausal transition is a huge shift in a woman's metabolic and hormonal health. It is a process where perimenopause blends into menopause. While the definition of menopause is 12 months without a spontaneous bleed, that is an artificial construct. In reality, it's a process of ovarian aging and hormonal decline where the early stage is often like a roller coaster of ups and downs rather than a steady decline.

In fact, right around perimenopause, many women will have a higher production of testosterone. The gonadotropin hormones alter, sending a signal to the pituitary gland, which in turn signals the ovaries. The luteinizing hormones and the follicle-stimulating hormones all change and the ovaries can no longer make the hormones they used to because there are no eggs. However, through all this, the ovaries may continue to produce testosterone, and women will often experience a *higher* sex drive temporarily. But then there is also the acne and the thinning of the head hair and the appearance of coarse hair on the chin—that's all testosterone!

The other thing that is happening at this time is some amount of atrophy in the vaginal area, which is called the genitourinary syndrome of menopause because it also involves the bladder. Bladder infections, urinary incontinence, and painful intercourse are all fallouts of this process as are hot flashes, night sweats, and sleeplessness. Sex drive also falters—after a period of higher sex drive, it dissipates.

Of course, different women experience menopause very differently, but the experience can be troubling for a lot of women. This is why I'm a huge advocate for hormone therapy in menopausal women. While treatment will not transform a woman into a 20-year-old, it will ameliorate some of the most troublesome symptoms to a significant extent. We cannot stop aging but we *can* slow it. We *can* postpone osteoporosis. We can improve quality of life, and we *can* improve sexual health and function. We don't want women to stop having sex at some point, but to continue to enjoy intimacy. Even women with atrophied vaginas can and do continue to have satisfying penetrative sex.

The decline of estrogen in the woman's body impacts the vascular system. It impacts the skin and makes it thin. The production of collagen, sebum, and other secretions decline, and basically, things dry up. This is why hormone therapy can make such a difference.

Things will be different but they can still be good

Sex among couples who are 50+ can be different since both men and women have experienced significant hormonal changes by now. Talking helps; it helps couples get through these things together. Maybe they can even share a laugh or two about what they are going through. Using lubricants and topical estrogen can ease the process. In some cases, seeing a pelvic floor therapist can help, as in the case of incontinence.

Spending time doing intimate things other than sex can help because it promotes bonding, which can be very meaningful for an older couple. Making a few adjustments can help a couple navigate the adventure of sexual aging and still enjoy good sexual health and function.

For optimal sexual health later in life, we also have to work to keep all our other organ systems in good health. As I have said repeatedly, it all ties in. If we continue with good foundational lifestyle choices, we can enjoy good sexual health and overall wellness for longer than we think.

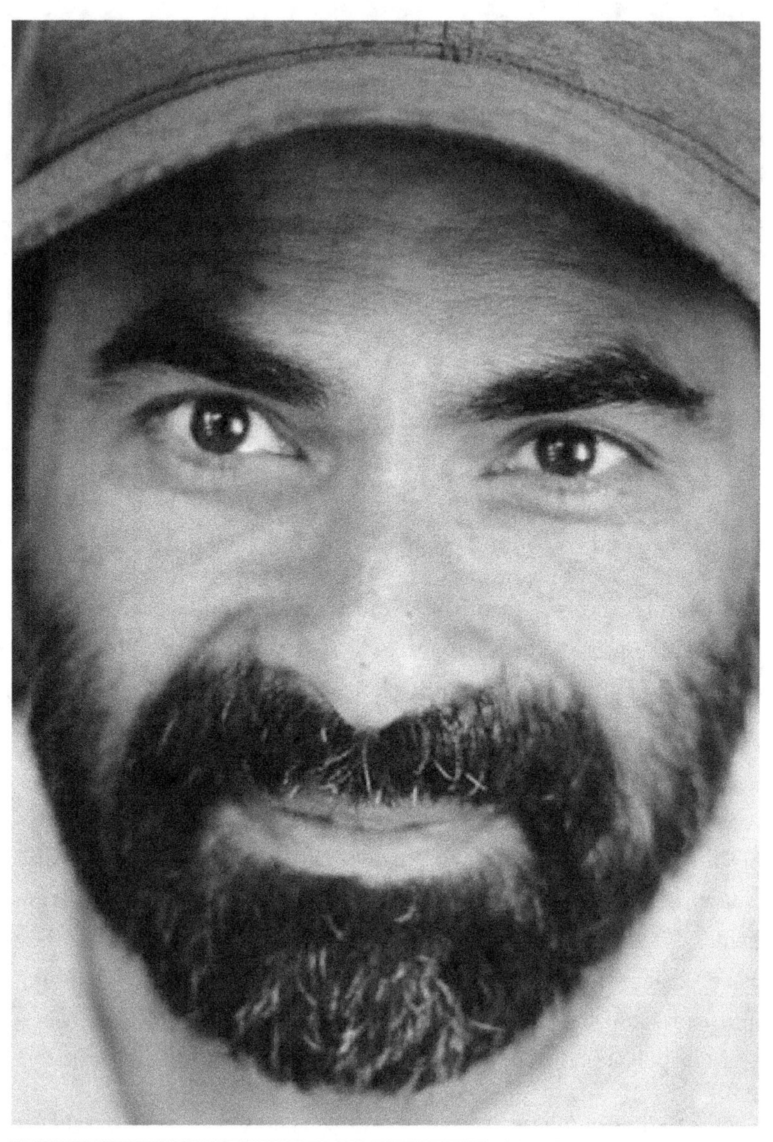

Navin Ramachandran

CHAPTER 3

Match.com revolutionized the world of dating. Suddenly people had access via the internet to others regardless of geographical constraints. There are many positives of the online dating world and there are also negatives. The dating scene changed and evolved, and app algorithms had an impact on this behavior. Tinder started out as an app for hookups but even that evolved to become a platform that users could use to forge meaningful relationships. It is important to know how dating websites work and how to remain safe while dating online.

MATCH.COM & OTHER DATING WEBSITES – HOW THEY CHANGED OUR WORLD

By Navin Ramachandran

It is kind of incredible to think that Gary Kremen and Peng T. Ong set up match.com all the way back in 1993 and launched it in April 1995. Those were the very nascent days of the internet, and online dating has come a very long way since then. Relationships that originate online are something we take completely in our stride today, but back in the mid-90s, this was probably an idea before its time. When we think back, it was actually very prescient to think about shifting dating online, where people could "meet" virtually and create meaningful relationships based on that.

Dating apps and websites have been able to connect people outside of the circumstances of work, outside of the circumstances of going to college together. They are able to connect people in the same town as well as in other towns to really come together. This is happening in a stressful world where busy lives leave little time for the kind of interactions that can lead to meaningful relationships. So, we could say that there have been many positive impacts of online dating.

On the flip side, there have been negative fallouts of connecting via the virtual world. It created a strange restlessness around dating. There is always the nagging thought at the back of the mind that there's something else out there that you're missing; could go for. This has probably created issues around commitment. We found that there is more of a churn in the space, where people are dating faster, for shorter durations. They are giving up on things a little faster—this I think is a potential significant effect of dating apps and websites.

Love in the time of COVID, and the problem of plenty

Even with all the dating websites around, there was still a lot of romance happening IRL. People were meeting on campuses, in offices, clubs and so on—and dating. Then COVID struck. People who were meeting at school, college, work, parks, bars, suddenly...weren't! According to studies, the lockdown literally rewrote the rules.[1] This confirmed what

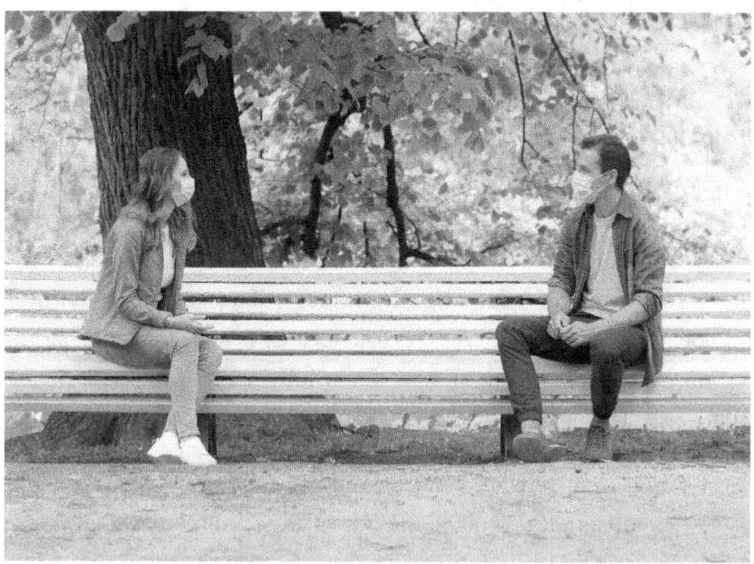

we already knew – that dating apps help to break down the "limits of physical and social disconnection, facilitating interactions between people with the promise of 'matching,' dating, and ultimately creating sexual or emotional intimacy."

This is not to say that online dating has not brought its own challenges with it. There is the problem of plenty, or rather the problem of choice.[2] People have the perception that there is potentially an endless supply of matches for them. It is something called the Paradox of Choice. In his book *Paradox of Choice – Why More Is Less*, psychologist Barry Schwartz speaks of how having too many choices can create anxiety. There has been a dramatic explosion in choice—from what toothpaste to use and what to eat for lunch, to whom to date and what professional decision to make.

Choice can become a problem instead of a solution. The sheer plethora of choices can be a problem. Studies have shown that when people experience choice overload (have more options than they desire) they can experience a "wide range of negative outcomes, from frustration and confusion, to regret, dissatisfaction, and even choice paralysis."

Then there is another problem: there could be users that are no longer subscribers, but whose profiles may still be available to view on the platform. Also, a lot of users create fake profiles simply by taking pictures off social media sites like Instagram and Facebook. So it is a good thing to remember that if something seems too good to be true, it probably isn't true.

Understanding how online dating works, and how it changed the dating scene

I am sometimes asked why it is that women tend to be inundated with responses while a man with a similar level of attractiveness may have far fewer responses. What we see is that this can differ significantly from region to region. In the New York region, women seem to outnumber male users whereas we see the reverse in a place like Anchorage, Alaska. Some dating websites also retain women's profiles even when they are no longer using the platform. This is in fact how Tinder started—

by getting attractive college women onto the platform as a way of attracting men. This is why we find that in a lot of markets, more men than women are seriously interested in dating.

When we think about it, online dating does have a very strong visual element, and studies have shown how men tend to respond more to visual sexual stimuli than do women.[3] This was actually another reason for Tinder becoming so popular versus match.com. On Match, users used to have to fill out a pretty long profile form. Women like to read these long profiles, and men tend not to. Tinder allows people to have very short profiles, the focus being on the picture rather than on what people write in the profiles. Men tend to swipe right first and filter other information later on. Obviously, attractive women get way more attention. The fact that women are so often inundated with attention was actually a turn off, and it is perhaps in reaction to that, that Bumble became so successful.

There is a general perception that online dating opened the door, so to speak, for a lot more people to have one-night-stands. Some organizations even claimed that online dating was pushing up the number of STIs. While exact data isn't readily available, it is true that dating apps increase people's chances of meeting—such as when someone was visiting a place for a few days and could line up a few dates for the duration of their stay. This wasn't possible earlier, so casual encounters of this sort have certainly increased.

One could also say that this has complicated the commitment issue somewhat – if, for instance, someone met a person while traveling and things really worked out. However, physical distance could now become a problem because one of those people has to return to wherever home is.

There is another complication caused by the fact that an app like Bumble could carry one's profile even when they delete the app. Now, the next time that a person logs in on the app, there will be a whole lot of messages waiting. All the attention may well encourage them to dive back into the world of dating, which they otherwise might not have done.

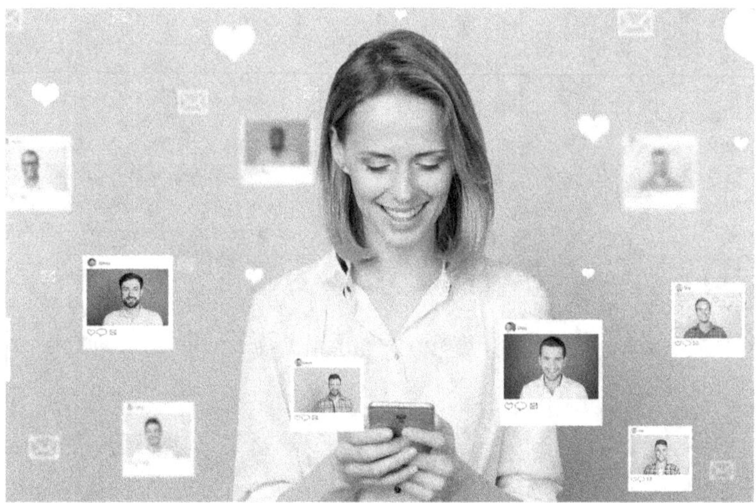

Here's an insight into the way some dating apps work: the algorithm makes an internal assessment of how attractive users on the platform are. Based on this assessment, the attractive members are going to be seen by a lot more people. This is a formula that works for many dating apps because of how it draws people onto the platform. While registration is free, the apps make money only if users opt for the paid subscription. One of the ways to convert registered users into paid subscribers is to give that illusion of having a lot of people interested in you. So a user is told that there are 10 people interested in you, but we will only show you one. If you want to see the rest, *pay for it*. Once converted, the app will try to keep them there for as long as possible because the lifetime value needs to be maximized for these people. That is how the system works.

Different strokes for different folks

Different people want different things from a dating app. While some focus on texting back and forth until they get a feel of the person, others may be in a hurry to meet. So how do we reconcile the one who likes to text, who may well be apprehensive about the other person wanting to meet, with the other type of person who might be fed up with all the texting? After all, people signed up to meet people, not to be pen pals. Not getting responses to messages, or all the back and forth texting can be frustrating for a lot of people.

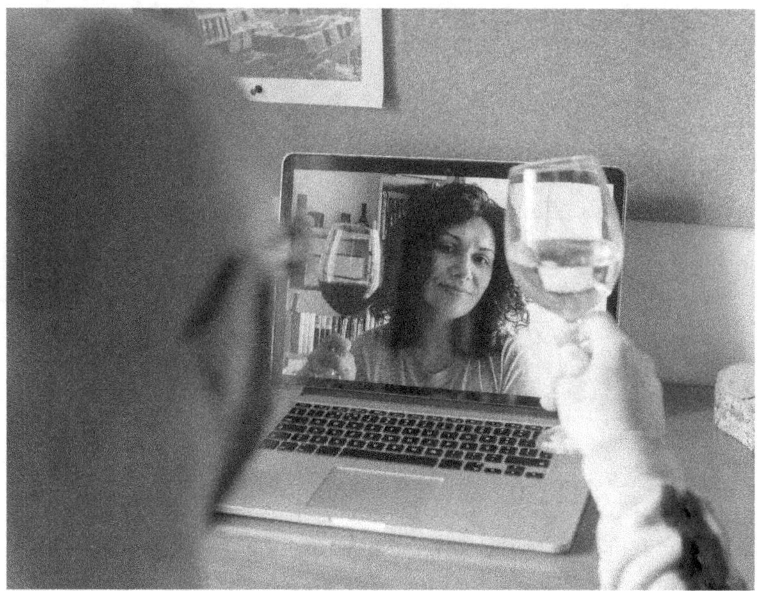

Another issue can be cultural differences. For instance, in a lot of cultures, physical intimacy at an early stage of a relationship is frowned upon, whereas among western cultures, the dearth of physical contact could be seen as a deal breaker.

When I came into Match Group, they had a strategic plan of combining offline dating and online dating. The idea was to have people meet at wine tasting events, go bowling, attend cooking classes. We thought to use the Match data to really get people to meet in person quicker for those inclined to do that. This strategy was largely abandoned after putting quite a bit of money into it. We found that when it comes to committing to a date and showing up to actually meet people, a lot of people are very hesitant.

At the time we had 400 events a month in different cities. We put the full force of the math behind this endeavor, but for a number of reasons, it didn't work. Firstly, there was that hesitancy about turning up for the event, which almost looks like a high school dance. People are awkward, and it can be difficult to align all the different kinds of energy people bring to the place. We also found that women would commit to these events, but men wouldn't. So these events would be 80% women and only about 20% men. So, trying to get a balance of men and women, for people who are interested in heterosexual dating, was difficult. We ended up having to cancel a lot of these events.

We saw how much of the time, women would huddle together at these events, and men would be on one side without talking to other men because they saw them as the "competition." With all the awkwardness and the strange dynamics of it all, these events didn't really work. And a lot of these people had signed up for the virtual, more indirect contact in any case, so why would they subject themselves to this social awkwardness?

Something else that we saw as online dating evolved is how TV was a big driver for people signing on to dating platforms. This was true in the late 1990s and the noughties. With the advent of handheld devices and the ubiquitous smartphone, TV lost its centrality in the scheme of things. For this reason, websites like eHarmony with its complicated matching system and difficult onboarding, lost out.

The Match Group also had a brief flirtation with speed dating. To begin with, the chairman of the Match Group was against speed dating, which was seen as not being aligned with the brand of the company.

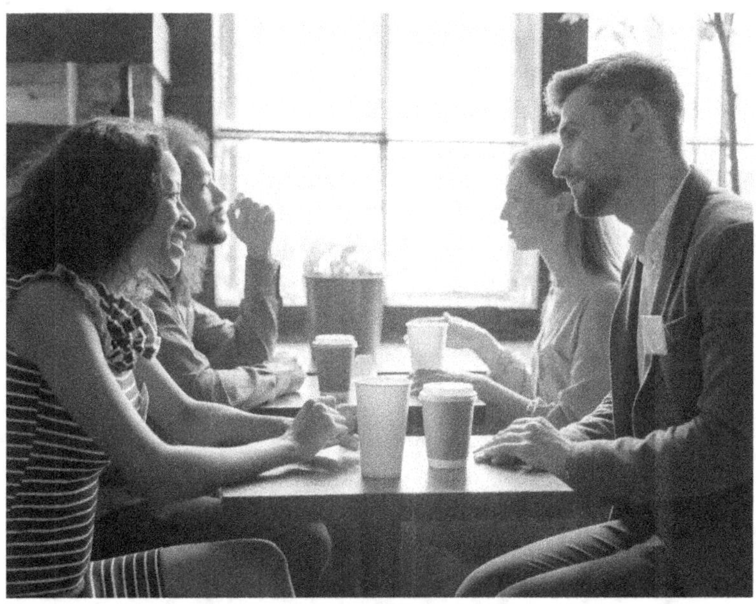

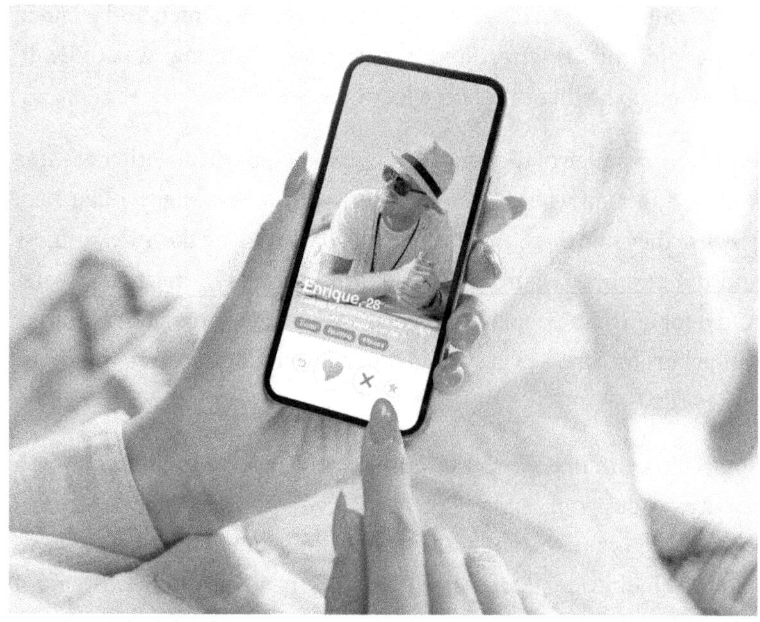

However, after attending these events and talking to singles all around the country, it seemed that America wanted speed dating.

I convinced management to actually try speed dating and we did roll out a whole bunch of speed dating events all over the US. While it worked to a limited extent, it didn't give the kind of returns we expected to the company. The costs just didn't justify continuing to do this in any big way. Initially, the theory was that once you have events, it will bring a whole new set of people into the Match Group and increase the size of the pie, which it really didn't do.

The age of Tinder and the formula for success

The swipe right functionality of Tinder was seen to become hugely culturally significant. Initially, it was seen as the hookup app, a place where people interested in sex could meet up. As with all such phenomena, this evolved with time. A few years after being set up in 2014, Tinder merged with the Match Group.

The whole hookup thing worked against and for Tinder. In the early days of Tinder, there was no advertising on Tinder. Typically, companies spend 30% of their revenues on advertising and marketing, but Tinder just grew without any of that. At one point Olympic athletes hooking up using Tinder was making a lot of headlines. This spurred more and more people to download and use Tinder. "For hookups" wasn't really a bad brand positioning for Tinder. It worked, but at the same time it was something that the management group wanted to veer away from. So the repositioning of Tinder as not just for hookups but for meaningful relationships was something that we felt was important to do at that time from a brand positioning standpoint.

I often get the question—*what is the formula for success in online dating?* Well for one, the picture matters! A good quality picture, preferably shot professionally, can make all the difference. It is your calling card. If the picture can show you as a nice person, a sociable person, a dog lover—all the better! This can determine the number and quality of inbound messages.

In general, make sure that the picture is not misleading or sending out the wrong message in any way. To the extent possible, be authentic— so maybe someone living in a tiny rented apartment shouldn't pose in front of a house with a swimming pool. In my experience, women will look at the details, but for a lot of men, the picture is the main thing. Also, avoid the "Where's Waldo" situation where one has to guess where you are in a picture with a bunch of other people.

Another tip: have a video chat, like a Zoom call with a person before you meet them in person. The chemistry with a person is completely different when you see them live on the screen. Getting a quick video interaction before meeting IRL is a really smart thing to do. At the very least, speak to them over the phone—even hearing someone speak can also give a lot of information.

Online dating has moved way beyond the CisHet communities and now caters to the LGBTQ community, as well as other niche groups with some very specific preferences. While apps like Grindr cater largely to the male gay community, about 10% of Tinder profiles are seeking out same-sex connections. However, for any such service, liquidity is key. You have to have enough users to be able to find a match that can actually work.

Geography does matter as well. Someone may not be conventionally attractive but could find a lot of like-minded people in, say, the San Francisco Bay Area. However, it could be very lean pickings in a more remote or non-urban location for such a person. This becomes even more important among niche groups. There is a dating site called Bloom that caters to kink and tries to connect people at kinky events and so on. People interested in meeting like-minded kinky people, often have to be prepared to travel long distances to an event or make more of an effort to make the connections they seek.

All this being said, there is actually a paucity of data to demonstrate how successful dating apps have been in matching people and helping create long-term relationships. How many end up in happy long-term relationships? How many couples get married? Some people send us pictures and letters, but mostly we have anecdotal information rather than substantive data. Also, from the point of view of a dating website, the idea is to continue to have subscribers on the platform for longer. So, from this standpoint, there is really no incentive to have people fall in love and have long-term relationships.

Choose a platform that aligns with your aims

Dating has changed a lot over the past few decades. I have friends who have been married for many years. Then after a divorce, when they put themselves out there again, they find that dating is *hard!* The world has changed and it can all be rather overwhelming. But then, things have changed for the better as well.

Dating is different, but it is also more efficient. Technology has ensured that there are so many more ways to meet people now. I would advise people to use the resources at their disposal. Examine the dating landscape and your goals; find the sort of dating app that aligns with your intentions. Are you looking just to get back into the scene, just to have a few dates, but you are not really serious about committing to someone? Choose the platform that optimizes for that. And if you're really looking for something long-term, go to the apps with fuller profiles and so on. There's such a wide array of options to choose from.

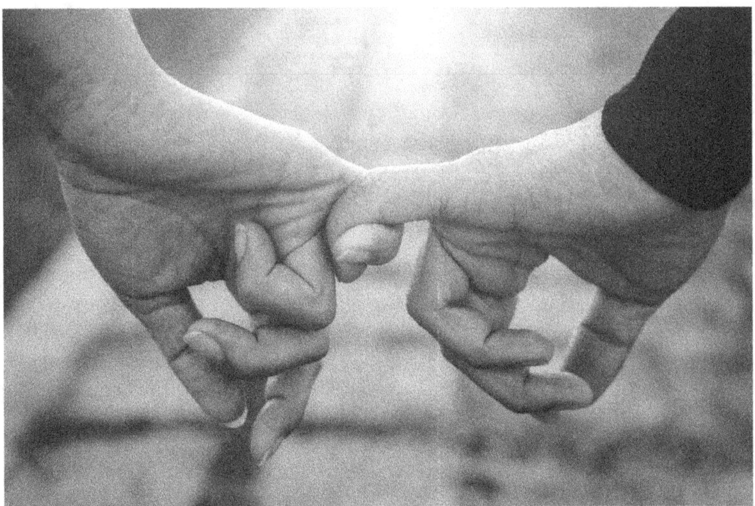

Also, remember that there are a lot of fake profiles on all of these dating sites, so just use caution. Being cat-fished where you trust people or as you're just wading back into online dating is very possible. So be cautious and just generally use your common sense.

Things have gotten easy—there are many choices and getting on to a platform is typically a simple process. However, many of these are apps that have hardly anybody on there. Dating is sort of universal and we all want to meet somebody and fall in love. This is so relatable to all of us that a lot of people think that they can start a dating company. There are a lot of people trying to get into that space, but few succeed because getting enough liquidity is incredibly difficult. Because of this, there's a lot of baiting being done to get people to pay for subscriptions. It can feel terrible to pay all that money and find no one interesting. At a time when one is just getting back into things later in life, this can be very dispiriting.

So, I would really talk to a few friends in your area that are also in the same situation. Ask them what apps they are using—for instance is Hinge better in this situation or Bumble? Where are the people you're looking for? Where do you find people in your age group? Ask a few questions. Only then will you know the kind of the liquidity in your area...and again, use caution.

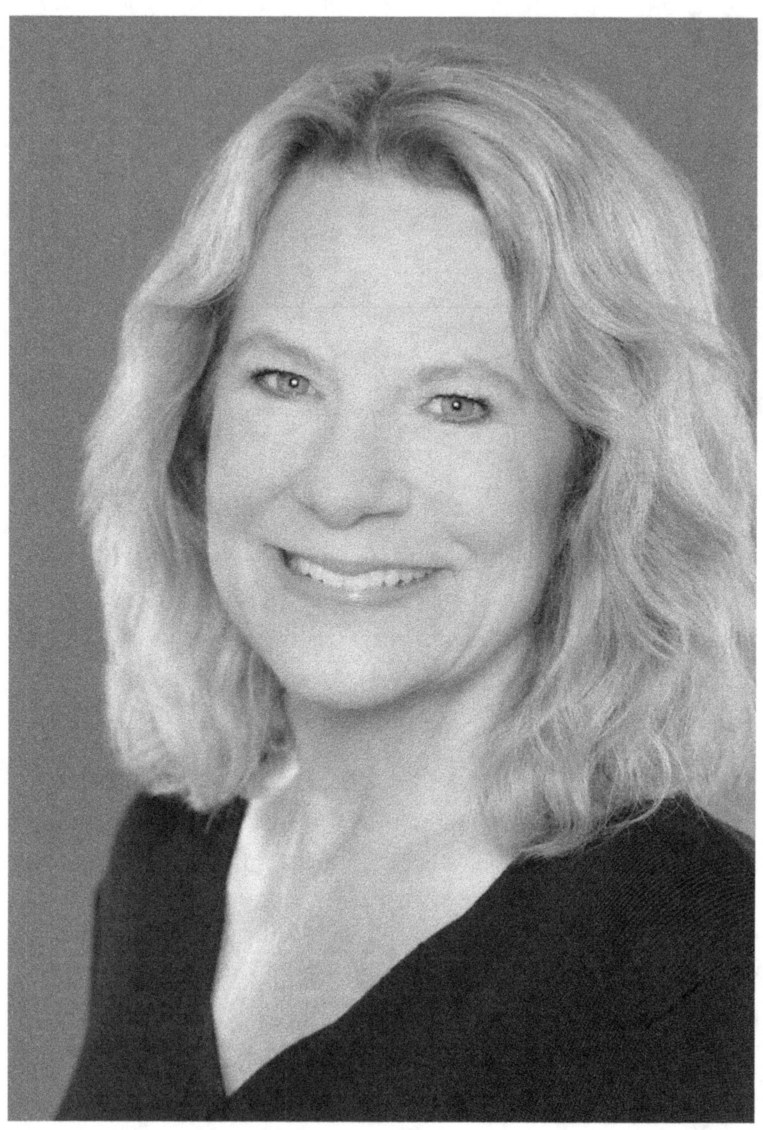

Dr. Vicki Matthews

CHAPTER 4

Good relationships are frequently the key to a successful and happy life. And this includes our sex life. Relationships are also a major predictor of our emotional and physical well-being. However, in the United States, we have over 40 million lawsuits a year, 50% of our marriages end in divorce, and the majority of our young adults are already in some form of relationship counseling. Clearly, it appears many of us have not yet figured out how to create good relationships. This needs to change because poor relationships not only impact our physical and emotional well-being, they do not support sexual wellness

CREATING HAPPY, HARMONIOUS RELATIONSHIPS

By Dr. Vicki Matthews

As motivational coach Earl Nightingale so accurately said, "Getting along well with other people is still the world's most needed skill." Wiser words were never spoken. Our relationships truly do impact every aspect of our lives.

From the moment we're born to the day we die, we navigate a host of relationships. As babies, we develop relationships with our parents and caregivers. As children, we forge relationships with family members, teachers, friends, and fellow students. As adults, we create romantic relationships as well as relationships with co-workers, neighbors, spouses, and children.

The degree of cordiality or friction in our every relationship can and will determine the quality of life we have, as well as our physical and mental well-being. Our relationships can elevate us or depress us, give us joy or plunge us into sorrow, and define or defeat us. And while we tend to think of relationships as unpredictable and capricious, in truth, it is very possible to predict which of our relationships will feel comfortable at every level—including sexually—and which ones won't. Even better, it is possible to improve every relationship we have by taking simple steps to understanding every relationship we have. And we can do this using the Five Elements model from traditional Chinese medicine.

The Five Elements model

The Five Elements model goes back millennia and is designed to explain the phases and interactions of different cycles. This can include the cycles of the seasons, the universe, or even a lifetime.

Acupuncture is based on the Five Elements model and uses specific techniques to shift energy patterns in our bodies to improve health and vitality. As I worked with the Five Elements model in my medical practice, I realized that our personalities are also based on the Five Elements. In very predictable ways, the Five Elements impact how we look at life as we move through the world. These different personalities can and will create different relationships. And the quality of these relationships will affect everything, especially our sexual wellness.

In my book, *The Five Elements of Relationships: How to Get Along with Anyone, Anytime, Anyplace,* I use this ancient Five Elements model to describe these five basic personality types—which I call Elemental Personalities—and the ways they automatically relate to one another. This information offers the opportunity to better understand everyone in our lives, enhance our relationships, improve family dynamics, and seek out people who will best support us in every conceivable way.

These five personality types are based on the elements in the model: Water, Wood, Fire, Earth, and Metal. Understanding these five different personalities is important because, in addition to helping us better understand the people in our lives, it helps us better understand

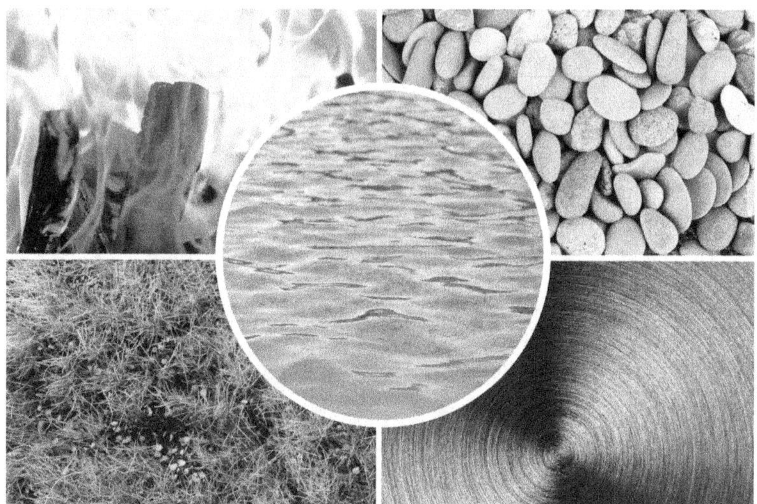

ourselves. Why is it hard for some of us to stay mellow and relaxed during stressful times? Why is quiet time by a fire pure heaven for some of us while others think a big party is the best thing in the world? Why are some of us workaholics and others could care less about a career? Why do process and protocol matter to some, while others love nothing more than just going with the flow? And why do we so often approach sex and sexual relationships so differently?

The quick answer to these questions is that while we all have all five of these elemental personalities in our energetic make-up, we are wired to lead with a specific one. The one we lead with is called our Primary Elemental Personality and affects everything in our life, including our stresses and our sexual wellness. An understanding of the Elemental Personalities provides important insights into how this works, so let's take a deeper look.

Water, Wood, Fire, Earth, and Metal

As mentioned, the Chinese conceptualized the elements based on the seasons. Water relates to winter and is focused inward. People with a primary Water personality are deep thinkers and often very creative. They enjoy philosophical discussions and books, and are usually happiest alone or with a few close friends. They almost always avoid crowds.

The Wood personality corresponds to spring. Wood people are the make-it-happen people who carry the energy of manifestation. Woods are visionaries who can see into the future, which makes them great planners. People with a primary Wood personality also love organization and accomplishment. Success matters a great deal to them, too, and they will frequently do whatever it takes to succeed.

Next is summer, a time of heat and activity. The personality that represents summer is Fire. With Fire personalities, there is usually a great deal of activity and lots of balls in the air. These personalities are full of fun, really like connecting with friends (old and new), and don't mind crowds or addressing a public gathering of thousands. They are outgoing people who thrive on attention, fun, and being with others.

Then we have Metal, which corresponds to autumn, when nature begins preparing for winter. Autumn represents a time for transitioning from outer manifestation to inner focus. People with a primary Metal personality love process and protocol. They love looking back and deciding what worked and what didn't, as well as what was necessary and what was not. They're the master discerners who, at the end of a season, decide what to release and what should go forward into the next cycle. They also love being asked their thoughts on any topic and will definitely have opinions.

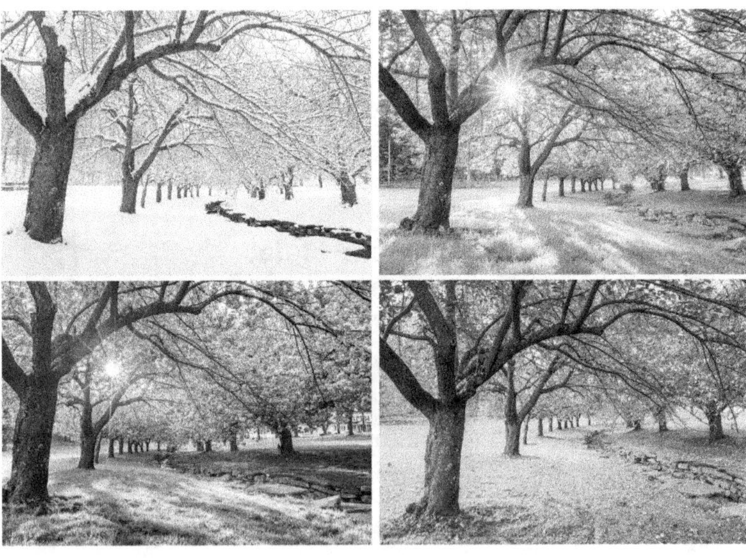

The last personality to discuss is Earth, which embraces balance and support. Earth energy manifests around the solstice and equinox times. The solstices are the times of greatest imbalance, when it's either mostly daylight (the long days around the summer solstice) or mostly night (the short days around the winter solstice). Earth energy supports balance. The equinoxes also relate to Earth's theme of balance. Both the spring and fall equinoxes are times of equal (balanced) day and night. People with a primary Earth personality love family gatherings, holidays, and food. They want everyone to be happy and are the ones who passionately value deep, lasting connections.

The Five Elements in relationships

When it comes to relationships, we might say that a Water personality could be good for a Wood personality because in nature, water feeds wood. But it isn't quite that simple with people. For example, one might think that a Fire-Water relationship wouldn't work well since water puts out Fire, yet that isn't necessarily so. Fires tend to go at top speed and sometimes literally do burn themselves out. Having someone there to help moderate their wild and crazy tendencies (douse their Fire) can be important.

The bottom line is that everyone can get along with everyone else if there is understanding. The Water person is going to have to understand that the Fire person needs activity, fun, and engagement to be happy, yet also needs balancing so they don't burn out. And the Fire person is going to have to understand that the Water person won't want to attend every wild party that comes along. Most of the time, they will be much happier at home reading a book. But even Waters need to enjoy the sun and fun, and no one can help them do that better than a Fire person.

Wood people focus on the future and can plan out exactly where they want to go. Metal people can assess the past to see what worked and what didn't. Fire people are instant connectors who do well as hosts, making public speeches or anything that requires interacting with strangers in a congenial manner. Earth people are the nurturers who make great parents and, given their love for food, are frequently great chefs. And Water people are the dreamers and creative types who can imagine anything and everything (but it will usually take a Wood person to make it happen).

That's the beauty of this model. The elemental personalities can all help build each other up, and they can also help moderate each other when necessary. That way, no one gets too out of balance.

Sexual wellness and the Five Elements

I define sexual wellness as a state of being that allows for physical, emotional, mental, and spiritual comfort regarding sex and sexual activities. This includes the ability to experience sexual pleasure, satisfaction, and intimacy when desired. The Five Element personalities will each manifest themselves in a specific sexual manner. This means that the primary elemental personality we are born with will have a direct impact on our sexual expression.

For example, a Water person is typically happy being alone. However, the sexual drive is wired into us all—it ensures the survival of our species, so the Water personality will also have sexual needs. But they may not care whether those needs are met by someone with whom they have a long-term relationship or someone they just met. For them, it's more a question of meeting their needs. This doesn't at all mean that the Water personality will always have casual sex. Yet there are times they may seek out people purely based on a need for intimacy and sexual expression.

A Wood person is likely to approach someone they are attracted to in hopes of taking the relationship to a certain place. That could be anything from a one-nighter to marriage. But because the Wood personality thinks of the future, they will most likely already have the desired end goal in mind. They could see sex as an aspect of intimacy, a necessary part of a relationship, a means to an end, or even a big win. But with a Wood, sexual expression will always mean something.

By definition, Fire people usually have very few boundaries. For them, life is about spontaneity, joy, and doing something that feels good. The Fire personality really enjoys social settings, dancing, and having

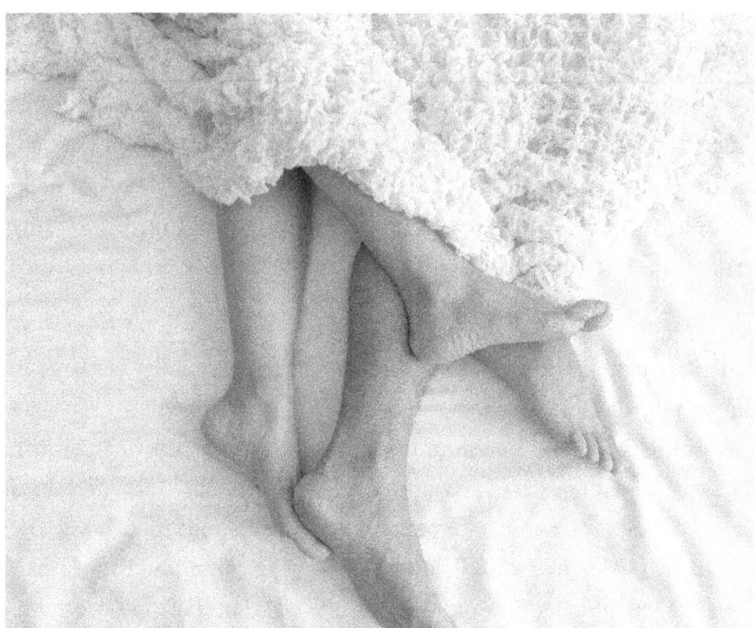

fun. And because they have fewer boundaries and less structure than the other Five Element personalities, sex can be a wonderful way for them to connect more deeply with anyone, almost anytime—if it feels right at the moment.

Metal people are fairly focused on themselves. While chemistry or compatibility are what might alert them to a relationship possibility, an urge to procreate or create a legacy may also be present. And for them, it could be as simple as, "This is what comes next in my life." That said, Metal people tend to be fairly picky. It isn't just about the sex. The Metal personality will usually assess the other person based on whether they are "right" for them and will be a benefit to their life. If so, they will usually move forward.

The Earth person focuses on supporting and nurturing other people. They also care deeply about children and family. This means that an Earth person, especially an Earth female, will often be attracted to sex more for the procreation aspect than for the excitement or pleasure of it. But once mated, most Earth people mate for life. For them, it is all about family, home, and connection.

It is important and useful to understand these five different personality types so that you can more easily understand yourself and the people in your life. The more you understand someone, the easier it is to get along with them. However, please remember that we each have all of these elemental personalities in our energetic wiring. And even though we have a primary elemental personality that we usually lead with, we can step into any of the other elemental personalities whenever we need them.

This means that while our primary elemental personality leads us in our day-to-day life, each of the other personalities will still impact how we live our life. For example, a person who is a primary Earth personality with a strong secondary Fire will probably want and need deep connections and excitement. It also means that their home life will likely be deeply fulfilling, and their sex life will probably be great. Because we all have Fire energy in us, it's a good bet that the more comfortable we are expressing the Fire part of our personality, the more robust our sexual encounters will be.

How our elemental personalities guide our sexual behavior

I was recently asked whether Water personalities, the people most inclined to be loners, might also be the personality with the fewest sexual encounters. My answer was, "It depends." While Waters are

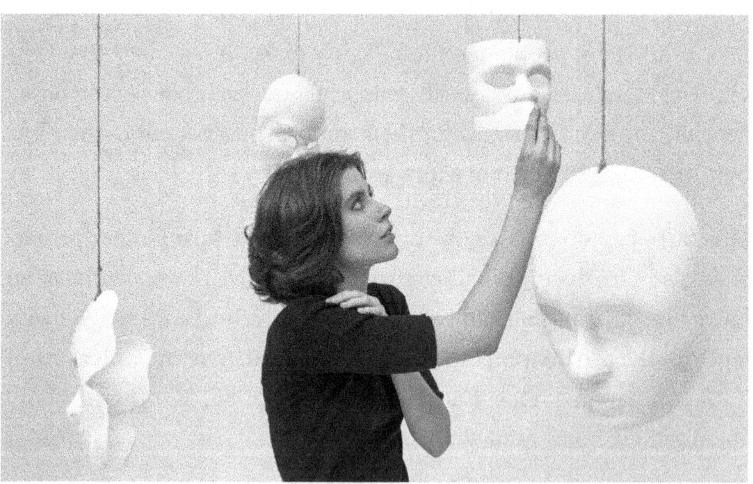

usually happiest alone or with a few close friends, as I mentioned before, the urge to procreate can be strong, even in a Water. If that happens, the Water person would likely tap into the Fire or Earth part of their personality and connect from there. That goes for all of the elemental personalities. We have them all and use them all at different times and for different reasons. And that includes around sex.

Here's a good example: The structured Metal personality will likely have a fairly methodical approach to sex, whereas a Fire personality is apt to be more spontaneous. Does this mean that a sexual relationship between a Fire and Metal is incompatible? It doesn't have to. But it does mean they will probably need to discuss expectations, desires, and needs.

The bottom line is that resolving sexual issues in a relationship often starts with understanding the people in the relationship and where major differences and disagreements lie. A couple could disagree regarding decision-making or finances. Or they could be thrown by day-to-day decisions like which babysitter to hire. Disagreements that linger can definitely impact sexual desire and activity. Once again, the point is that compatibility and connection begin with understanding. And the Five Elements excel at helping us understand each other.

For instance, as a primary Wood personality, I don't care that much about detail and rules, but they matter very much to my Metal husband, so we honor that in our marriage.

Accomplishments, milestones, and getting things done matter more to me, and he honors my priorities (for the most part). So, to get along with someone, I believe we have to understand the person we're with and what matters to them. The better we understand them, the better the relationship—and the sex—will be.

Enhancing sexual wellness in life

When our energies and personalities are balanced, we manifest the best version of ourselves. If we are out of balance, we are unable to manifest anything very well. So, what can we do to improve sexual wellness?

The first step is self-care and maintaining balance in life. For example, it's possible for personality elements to reduce interest in sexual activity without any obvious or external cause. Suppose a Fire person is born into a strictly religious or conservative family. As they mature sexually, they may naturally lean towards behaviors that could be deemed inappropriate by their family. If they want to dance and party, and that is frowned upon by their family, the Fire person will be unable to fully express themselves. This can (and usually will) create a situation where their Fire energy is diminished because they didn't have the avenue of expression that is most important to Fire: connecting with people in a fun way. But as they consciously work to increase the expression of their Fire, they can and will regain balance.

Being true to oneself is important; it helps balance and restore our energy. People with sexual issues must look at themselves first. Do they frequently have unbalanced emotional expressions like jealousy, anger, panic, or fear? This can indicate that their primary elemental personality is out of balance.

When I meet with couples, once I determine their primary personalities, I can assess their likely sexual chemistry with some degree of accuracy. Very often, a lack of sexual chemistry is due to an aspect of someone's personality that is uncomfortable with sex for some reason. We then work on helping the couple balance (and understand) their elemental personalities and how they best relate. As their understanding grows, sex usually becomes a welcome expression for both of them. It goes without saying that we need to be comfortable with the expression of our sexual energy to have sexual wellness. The more comfortable we are around this energy, the more comfortable we are around sex, and the better sex is!

That said, staying balanced physically, emotionally, mentally, and spiritually is also going to help keep sexual energy and all of our energies balanced. I discuss a great deal more of this in my book, *Five Elements of Relationships: How To Get Along With Anyone, Anytime, Anyplace.* It covers ways to balance and realign our essential personalities and is available on Amazon and Barnes & Noble. My book also has dozens of ways to build and balance Fire energy. And while not specifically covered in the context of sex, everything in there about building and balancing Fire energy will absolutely work to improve sexual wellness.

I also do sessions with couples and individuals across the globe. I can help them understand their elemental personality—there is actually a quiz on my website that helps people determine their elemental personality—and then we can work through the issues that they face, including sexual ones.

When I start to work with people, they quickly realize that they pretty much already understand all five of the elemental personalities. That's because we all have Waters, Woods, Fires, Earths, and Metals in our lives. When I describe an elemental personality, people will often realize, "Oh my gosh, that's Mom!" or "That's my boss!" Anytime we can stop and really consider the people we relate to, we come to better understand them. That's when relationships can improve, and we really can get along with anyone! I know this for a fact because it happened to me.

I like to tell the story (from a long time ago) of the time my husband of two weeks refused to exceed the speed limit in the desert—a place where there was literally no one but us. It made me question if I even liked him. It took me a while to understand why he'd do this (he follows the rules, I usually don't). But once I understood him, I started to like the guy I loved because I understood the guy I loved.

If you understand the person you love, the child you have, your boss, or the people that you're training—if you can understand them and their behaviors—what seems annoying suddenly makes sense. And with this understanding, we can create healthy relationships. The truth is that anytime sex is part of the relationship, the best you can do to create sexual wellness is to understand—truly understand— the person you are relating to. From there, magic happens!

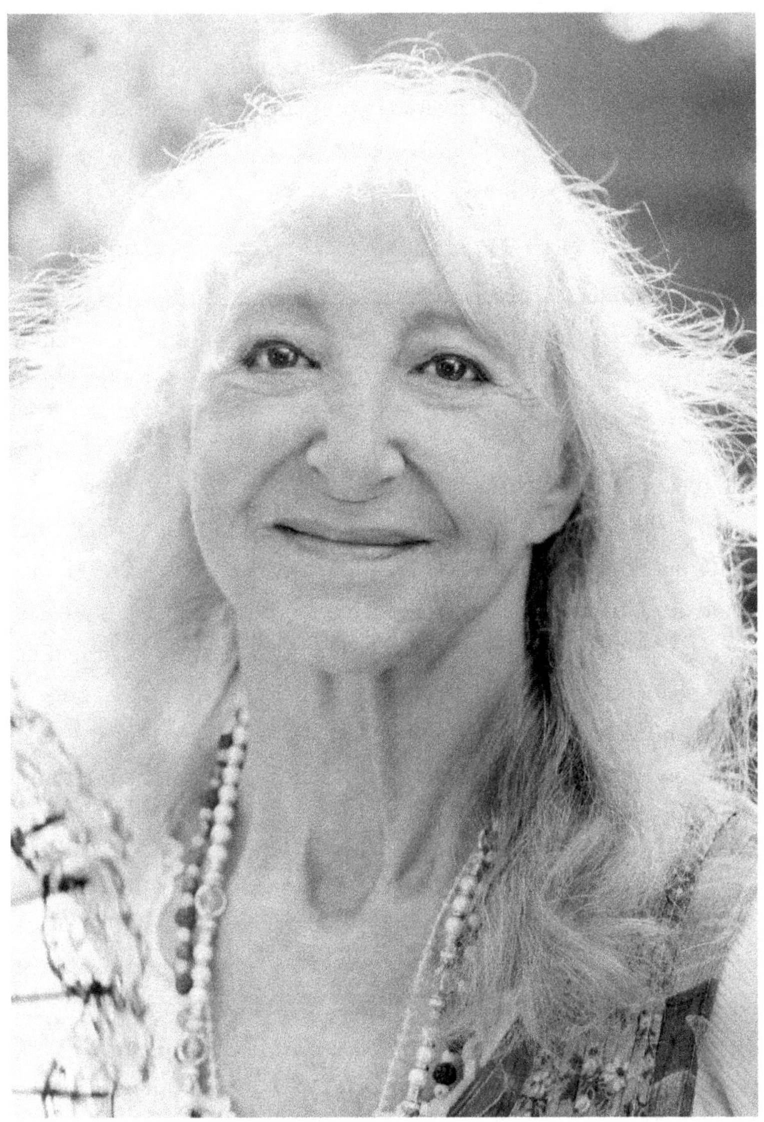

Margot Anand

CHAPTER 5

*There is a close connection between sex and spirituality.
Buddha taught us to be without desire when one is full of desire.
This leads to a state of nothingness that transcends not only
desire but also all types of suffering. It is possible to create sensory
awakening rituals that not only enhance the act of sex but also
strengthen one's relationships and help one experience ecstasy.
When one is able to experience true ecstasy, that is like shaking
hands with divinity. It is true freedom, which opens a person up to
a host of possibilities and to their own creative potential.*

THE ART OF BEING DESIRELESS AT THE HEIGHT OF DESIRE— WHAT THIS MEANS AND WHY IT'S IMPORTANT

By Margot Anand

I had the opportunity to meditate for 20 days—silent meditation in an incredible place—set up just for advanced meditators in the jungles of Bali. I had my own schedule of meditating with beautiful flowering plants all around: meditation in the morning, then yoga, then breakfast, then spiritual conversations around Dharma. I studied Buddha as well as more modern masters such as Osho, and read commentaries on the Heart Sutra and more.

All of this led me to create my own meditation method. I was able to actually transcend the mind and body. I was, at one point, a disabled woman that hobbled around on a cane. I corrected myself. I'm now pain-free. I can sit on a pillow and fly in an infinite space of silence.

In this state of awakening, we become one with all that is…we exit our personality, our ego, our mind, and our thoughts. Buddha taught us about transcending suffering, and the kind of attachments that cause suffering. It is desire that creates craving and then addiction and then suffering—as in the case of someone like Jeffery Epstein who indulged his sexual cravings and ended up addicted.

So to avoid that suffering, we need to create that sense of equanimity. We must strive to be *desireless at the height of desire*. That's the insight that I, Margot Anand, am sharing with you! This means that you are so totally present in the moment that you don't know what the next moment is going to bring. That is the only way not to suffer; to simply let go and not to be caught up in desire. The idea is to achieve equanimity via relinquishment and letting go, which brings us into a neutral state beyond the goal-oriented attitude of desire towards an object of pleasure.

"Love What Is"

Now as I prepare for my eighties, a new decade of life here on Earth, I find that as we get on in years, it becomes very, very important to prepare ourselves for that final exit. There are two exits: one is the exit of the mind or spirit: this is the awakening. The other is the exit of the body, which is death.

In all things, equanimity, being fully present in the moment is vital. As Byron Katie so beautifully expresses in her book, *Love What Is*. When we are in equanimity, we are ready for anything. We don't desire things to be this way or that way. We don't want our reality to follow our mental script, and we don't want to defend our personality. The ego is no longer important and we give ourselves over to the here and now. We are, in a way, empty-minded. This is not a negative thing; it merely means that we are in a state of perceiving and witnessing. That witnessing factor is very important.

What I learned during my 20 days of silent meditation is difficult to condense, but I recommend that people study Buddha's teachings about how to transcend suffering. His teachings actually meet the

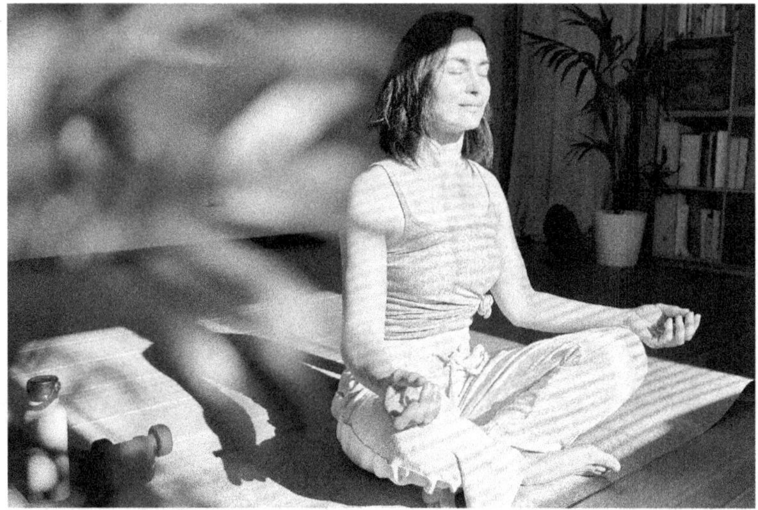

discoveries of quantum physics. I would urge people to make contact with their environment. We have feelings and sensations: we feel hot, we feel cold. Then we have perceptions via the synapses in the brain. We interpret these and translate these into a qualitative opinion, good or bad, etc. These patterns of feeling, perceiving, and interpreting have been ongoing since birth.

Practicing meditation

Meditation helps us transform or change these patterns of perceiving and interpreting. It enables us to move through those emotions— negative and positive—and to realize that we as human beings are ecstatic beings, sovereign beings. We are free, full of light; we are blissful. In that state of bliss, sex is not important. *Nothing* is important when we realize that we're free; that we are with God/Goddess, that we *are* the divine.

Most frequently, I have people sharing their difficulties with meditation: the mind wavers, or there is an interruption, or one gets distracted. It is actually quite simple to overcome these issues for anyone who wants to meditate. You have to talk to your mind. Your mind is in your service. It is your friend. You have to thank your mind for being there for you. You then forbid the mind. You forbid any thoughts or memories from the past, or projections from the future.

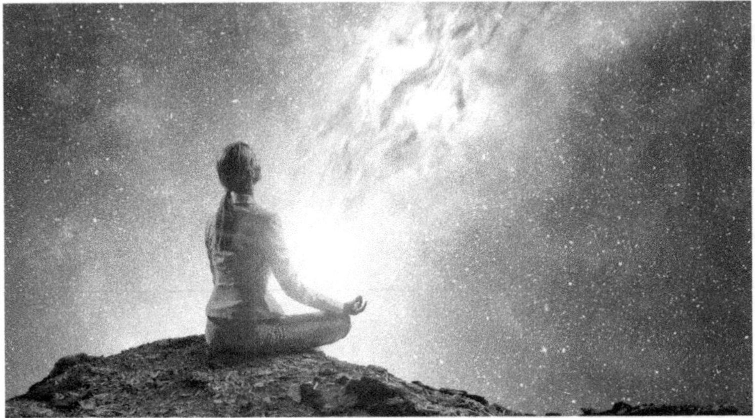

You have to have this internal dialogue with your mind in order to steady it and calm it. You cannot watch your breath and watch your thoughts at the same time. Sex is like this. If you want to enhance your sensations during sex, you have to develop the three keys to ecstatic orgasmic bliss—breathing, movement, and sound—which form a part of my training modalities.

Sex and spirituality

I have been steeped in the ancient concept of Tantra for decades, so I often get the question: *what is Tantra?* Tantra is an ancient concept drawn from Buddhist and Hindu traditions, and it means weaving the many contradictory aspects of our personality into one whole, into oneness. It brings together many realities to help expand your consciousness. Tantra is the science of enlightenment as laid down in the ancient scriptures. It has been around for thousands of years and has recently seen a revival.

For instance, my friend Lorin Roche revives an ancient 15th-century text in his book, *The Radiance Sutras*, a dialogue between Lord Shiva and his consort Shakti. Shiva and Shakti speak about 112 gateways to enlightenment in a very central, real, connected, poetic way. This puts the ancient tradition in a more modern context that we can relate to.

I have been among the first to shine a light on Tantra in the West, and have been speaking about the teachings of Tantra since the 1970s with specific reference to sexuality. I ask people to be aware—to choose with awareness, to ask what brings them joy and what doesn't. Are they doing something out of duty or because it brings pleasure? When we choose with awareness, it opens the door to the spirit.

Cultivating orgasmic energy

You could say an orgasm a day keeps the doctor away. Apart from the purely physical aspect, we can also cultivate orgasmic energy. You do this by plucking the feeling of vibrational excitement, and by channeling it through the energy centers connected to the endocrine glands. The energy courses through the central channel of the body all the way to the crown.

We can expand consciousness beyond the boundaries of the body into all that is: into oneness with the universe. This is the point where everything feels perfect. This sounds crazy considering what an imperfect world we live in. However, perfection can be a state of mind. It can be something we can achieve if we can reach that inner source. And that's what Tantra is about: transmutation of sexual energy into bliss.

In my book *The Art of Everyday Ecstasy*, I explain how bliss circulates through each of the chakras, and how each of the chakras have certain behaviors associated with them. We need to direct that bliss to the crown, because that's where freedom is. If a woman can do that, she doesn't depend anymore on the style of lovemaking of her partner. She doesn't have to depend on whether her partner lasts an hour or five minutes, because she's plugged into her own source of energetic expansion.

When I work with couples, I work with each person individually so they can learn to open their central channel to bring pleasure through the chakras. The couple then comes together in a process I developed, called the yoga of pleasure. This is the ideal situation where the man's first chakra is positive and active: it's Yang. The woman's first chakra is receptive, and she is Yin to his Yang. The two connect automatically, and one feeds the other to start a circle of energy between the two and inside each individual. I teach this in my training and also speak about it in my book, *The Art of Sexual Ecstasy*.

We teach all of this in our Love and Ecstasy training at our Skydancing Tantra Institutes, which, by the way, are the only ones in the West that have existed for 35 years. We offer our tremendously popular Love and Ecstasy (LET) training course called *Sky Dancing Tantra*. We have institutes in the United States, France, Switzerland, and Germany. Information about this is available at skydancingtantra.org, and people can join individually or as a couple.

Self-awareness and sex

One of my teachers, the mystic Osho, used to say this, "When a woman and a man come together in the bedroom as lovers, they aren't just a woman and a man, but also the father and mother of the woman, and the father and mother of the man." By extension there is also the presence of the grandparents, uncles and aunts here. This is especially true in India, where people live in extended families and a person marries not just another individual but their entire family. Everyone in the family will have an opinion on the couple, which can influence the lovers to behave in a certain way.

It is vital to be more meditative about understanding the power of the sacred and the delicacy of love, and to proceed slowly to integrate sex with the heart and the soul. This is not easy because we're always in a hurry in this society. We tend to look at the orgasm as the goal, but that doesn't work because the woman and the man have different ways of reaching it. If the partners approach this in a conscious, awakened manner, setting aside the ego, they have a much better chance of reaching an expanded state of consciousness together.

Now don't get me wrong – good sex is good sex and we need not undervalue this. A married couple can become bored with each other over time, and the sex may no longer be as good as it used to be. I have worked with couples like this to go beyond the good sex, to expand the experience. There is a discipline in tantric practice, things that couples can focus on to enhance the experience, as my books and my programs teach.

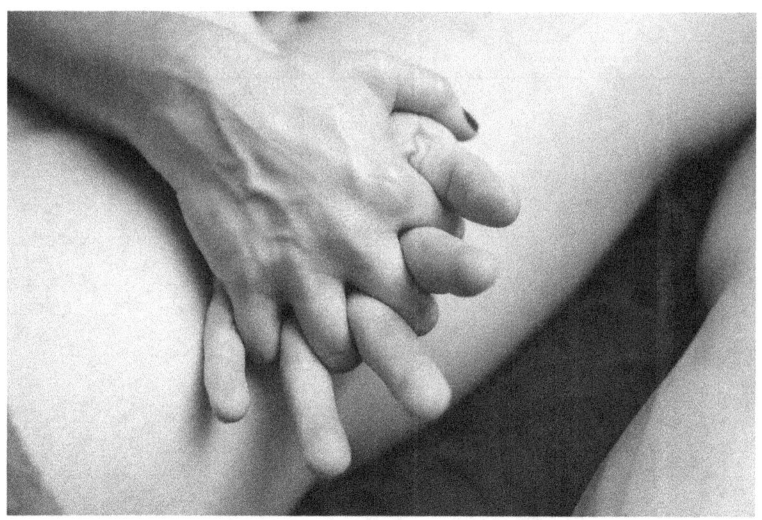

Orgasm need not be the only goal

So while the sex is important, in western societies there is perhaps too much emphasis on penetration and the male orgasm, possibly because of the evolutionary need to propagate the species and because of religious beliefs. We need to look beyond this. Several people have spoken about it, such as the Taoist master Jolan Chang. In my view, a man's age and health are important factors. If a man is feeling tired or sick, he should retain his seed and not let go of it. So there is merit to semen retention[1] as disciplines such as Ayurveda have demonstrated.

Speaking personally, in my life I have often had two lovers and this is something I will recommend to all women (though something that our puritanical society will frown on). While one of my lovers was a tantric master who promoted retention, the other one was a Reichian therapist. And true to Wilhelm Reich's perspective, orgasms that include as many ejaculations a day are good and possible. If a man releases all the time, he gives his power away. If a man wants to really hold his power, he should train as a tantric lover. This gives him the power to take pleasure in coming to *almost* the point of no return before pulling his energy back effortlessly. All the while he stays relaxed through each of his chakras to expand his consciousness. It makes him the captain of his ship, which is what I recommend.

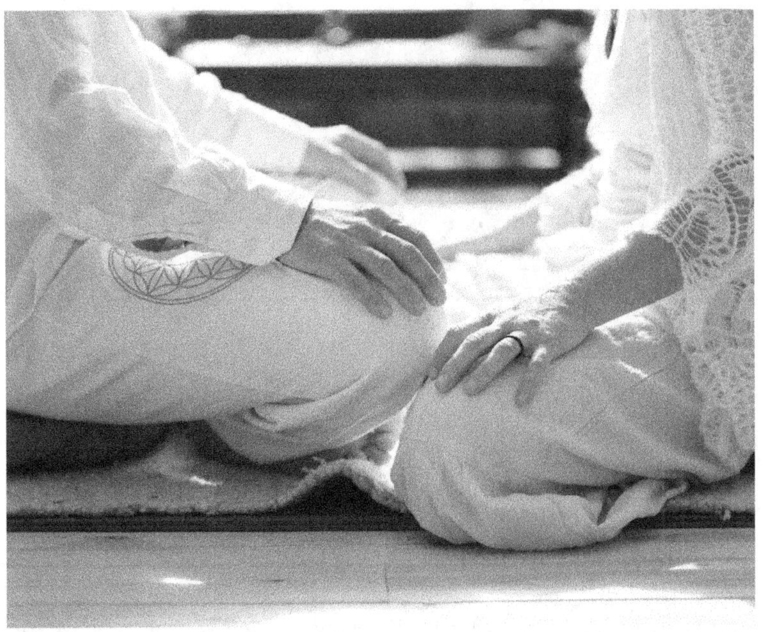

It can be more difficult for a man, but retaining release can be pleasurable. Men can practice something that I call sexual breathing: lying down, with the knees up and feet flat on the floor, there is a slight rotation of the pelvis, and then a slight tightening of the perineum area (between the sex organ and anus). Inhaling with the pelvic movement, the man pulls the energy to the first chakra, the second chakra, and so on. It can be timed with some jazz music to make that pelvic movement sexy! Doing this for five or ten minutes a day will open a central channel in the body. This can easily be applied to lovemaking. It helps tamper down the speed and the excitement so that it becomes a kind of erotic dance with one's partner. It can be frustrating to begin with, but men find that the body responds positively to the pressure.

I have seen how my body responded positively—at one point I was walking with a cane but now I'm completely healthy. I'm nearing 80 but I am healthy and fit, so anyone can do it, if they decide to do it. *You choose with pleasure*—one of the reasons I'm in Bali and not in America! We have that sexual power in us, which we need to awaken and not abandon. The language of love is like learning a sport or a new skill—we persevere until we learn how to do it.

Orgasm and the woman

A woman is not depleted by orgasm, even multiple orgasms. She can channel her energy in the orgasmic response. Where she does lose energy is during her period. So orgasm itself is not the issue, but the timing of it can be. Men are faster, women need more time. A woman can aim for as many orgasms as possible and can achieve this by moving energy through her chakras. This is good for her endocrine system and even for her sense of humor! If she is fulfilled, she is going to create less drama in her life, and she is going to be generally more relaxed.

It isn't about finding the right man or about getting him to do what she wants. It is more about a woman working on herself to open her channels, about taking care of herself, and being more open to lovemaking and more orgasms.

Now whether it is LGBTQ people or people having multiple partners, it is about finding ways to be fulfilled and at peace with oneself. This is no one else's business. The French believe that if a leader has a wife and then also a mistress, it is no business of the public to question that. If this sexual fulfillment is what it takes for one to be an effective leader, then the public has no business disapproving. This was true for my own parents where my mother knew about my father's other lover. In this process, it is all about practicing the union of two halves, yin and yang, receptive and emissive.

My secrets to the ultimate love life

I train people to look for and find their sensory awakening. In my book, *The Art of Sexual Ecstasy*, I explain some of the tantric lovemaking techniques of the East to my readers in the West to help them create life-affirming, sex-positive attitudes. It isn't just about achieving better and longer orgasms but also about healing and strengthening relationships.

In my book, *The Art of Sexual Ecstasy*, I explain the importance of creating a sensory awakening ritual. It can be something like giving one's partner a surprise, asking one's partner for an hour of their time, then blindfolding them, and then initiating the ritual. It can be a great turn on and later, the recipient of the ritual turns into the giver. This may not necessarily be sexual, but can still be deeply intimate and affirming for a couple.

When they experience ecstasy, human beings open up to their full potential. They have, in a way, shaken hands with the divine, and are facing the fact that they are sovereign beings that can connect directly with the universe. There is no interlocutor and no priest; just a direct connection with our divine source. Governments and religions don't want this; they don't want independent individuals that make their own decisions and are the creators of their own destinies.

There is no need to be bound by the dictates of any government or religion. You can explore the entire world to find the path that is yours, the vocation that is yours. This is why so many Americans are giving up their jobs. They don't want to be automatons doing as they are told all the time. They want to be free to decide for themselves. When you are in that space, you become truly free, and infinite possibilities open up.

What is next for me?

I have in the past been a coach to Hollywood stars. I have been asked to teach at the Kennedy School of Political Leadership at Harvard because many leaders needed to learn how to channel their sexual energy. However, that was about feeding the ego and I am no longer interested in that. I no longer want to dedicate any energy to cultivating and protecting the ego. This is not me, you are not you, and we are all illusion—Maya. This is the point when I am more interested in other realities and curious to know more about what I can do and where I can reach.

While in the process of writing this, I plan to go off on a 30-day silent meditation retreat in the jungle. Then I want to go sailing with friends. I want to sing and have fun. I plan not to teach, though this is difficult because more workshop ideas keep coming to me. I want to see what emerges further along my spiritual path.

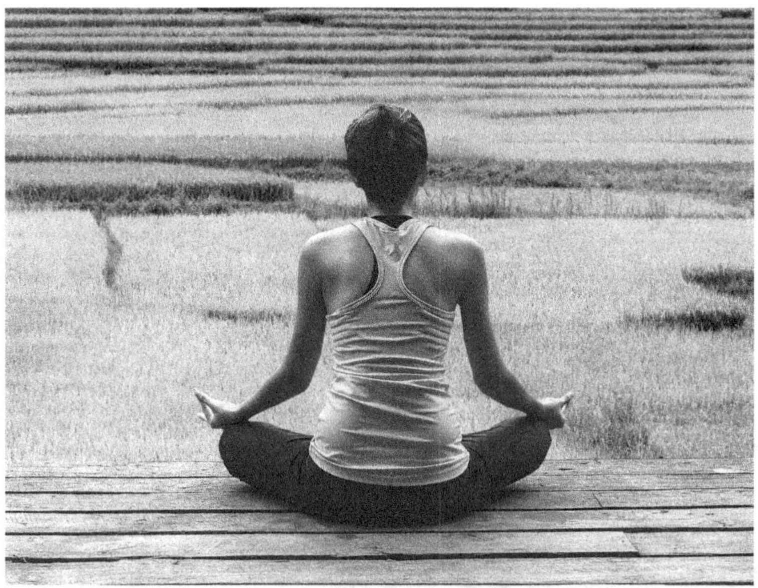

A friend pointed out to me that I seem to be having fun all the time, and they are not incorrect. I feel that when one has achieved a certain degree of awakening, one achieves a stabilized contentment. We create a certain connection with source consciousness and there is really no reason to be unhappy. We can choose not to be trapped in the little details of life, and grow in ways that include laughter and humor because this is what opens up the heart!

I would recommend some books for further reading to my readers. First is *Mindfulness, Bliss, and Beyond,* which is a meditation book by Ajahn Brahm where we learn not only about "mindfulness" but also about "kindfulness"; where we add another dimension to the process of meditation. In the book *Passionate Enlightenment,* Miranda E. Shaw speaks about the foundational role of women and dakinis in the unfolding of Tantric Buddhism as a spiritual path for men and women to follow and practice to experience awakening together. She also argues in favor of and presents evidence of the female founders of tantric traditions and rituals. So go ahead! The time has come in this world, to promote the victory of the light—to find your freedom, claim your ecstasy, and share it with others.

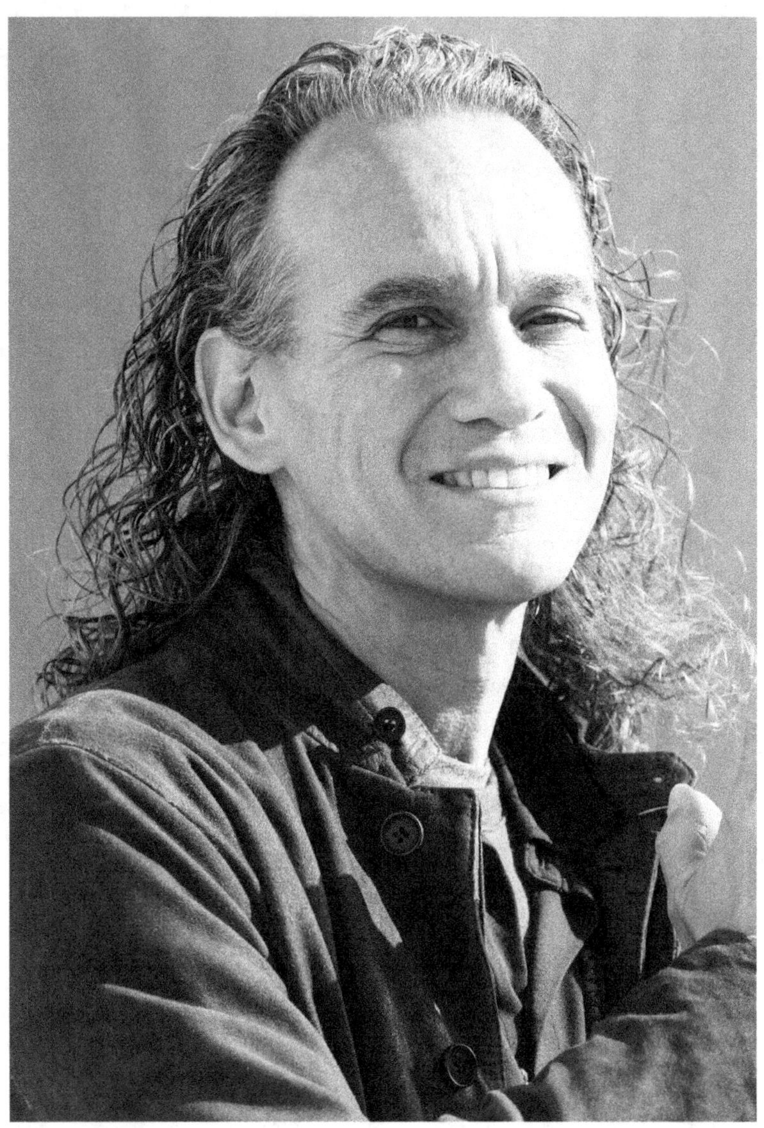

Ulises Calatayud

CHAPTER 6

We tend to think of Tantra as being about sexual prowess; however, it is much more than that. Tantra is the very warp and weft of life, and can be applied to every moment to make life happier and more meaningful. There is no good or bad here—we must embrace what comes naturally to each of us. We can use traditional techniques, breathe in specific ways, and create visualizations to bring about healing—all to free up the chakras in the body, create sexual energy, and harness our inner potential.

TANTRA IS ABOUT MORE THAN JUST SEX—IT IS THE TAPESTRY OF LIFE ITSELF

By Ulises Calatayud

My conscious walking in the path of Tantra began with a searching, a seeking for something more, something beyond a successful career as an international executive in the corporate world. I started with meditation and breathing techniques. I started to engage very actively and very intensely, looking for that spark to light it up. This quest has taken me along many fascinating paths and has been a rewarding journey that is still ongoing.

I used to move around a lot during my life in the corporate world— I went from city to city, wherever my company and my work took me. All the while, I was engaged in intense learning and practice of meditation and breathing with my teacher. At one point, I moved to New York City and continued to practice, mainly on my own. Back then, I left a whole bunch of audio cassettes and a little tape recorder with my teacher. He would record the classes and mail me those cassettes. I would listen and practice from 4:00 AM to 6:00 AM each day—and this is how I got started on the path that leads to the present moment as a teacher of yoga, Tantra, and more.

The world of Tantra

At the time I could see the changes that were happening to me: the physical, mental, and spiritual changes. However, I was missing that sense of community. I would occasionally meet my teacher in Mexico City, but there was still that yearning for a community. I was also looking to reconcile the connection between my meditative and breath techniques, and the sexual energy that I felt. How could I keep learning and progressing?

For a while I contemplated celibacy—was that the way to go? I grew up in a Catholic environment where sexuality was always shrouded in secrecy; a taboo subject never spoken about. My meditation teacher also never spoke about sexual energy. In most traditions, sex and sexuality tend to be overlooked or avoided. However, I always felt that this was a big part of wellness; a part of the human experience that we all needed to explore and embrace more fully.

My serendipitous meeting with Margot Anand

It was by sheer serendipitous luck, or coincidence if you like, that I came to be associated with Margot Anand. Back when I was working in NYC, one day I was near a place called the Open Center in New York City. I chanced upon a Tantra workshop. I felt that here, finally, I might find some of the answers that I sought for my sexual energy. Here, perhaps, I would find the community that I was looking for. So I enrolled in this class that I would take over the coming weekend.

However, even before that weekend could roll around, something else happened four days before. On my way to the train home from Midtown in New York City, I had a piece of paper handed to me. The piece of paper had a quote from one of Margot Anand's books. Below this was a time and an address. That address was half a block from where I was and the time was 15 minutes from the time on my watch. I read the quote about being in an ecstatic mode all the time, and I thought of the magic of time and space! I was transported to an ecstatic mode—it was meant to be!

So I called home and said I would not make it for dinner. I went to the address at the given time and I sat and listened to this beautiful woman speak. Every word was amazing to me, I was already finding some of the answers I sought. I found myself saying, "Wow!" The lady next to me said, "Isn't she amazing?" And I agreed! The lady asked whether I had read any of Margot's books, and I confessed I hadn't. So what was I doing at what happened to be a book signing? Like I said, serendipity!

Later I got a book and lined up to get my book signed. When I finally reached Margot, I asked for her phone number. When she looked at me quizzically, I said, "I want to learn from you." She invited me to attend one of her retreats, one that was starting on that very Friday.

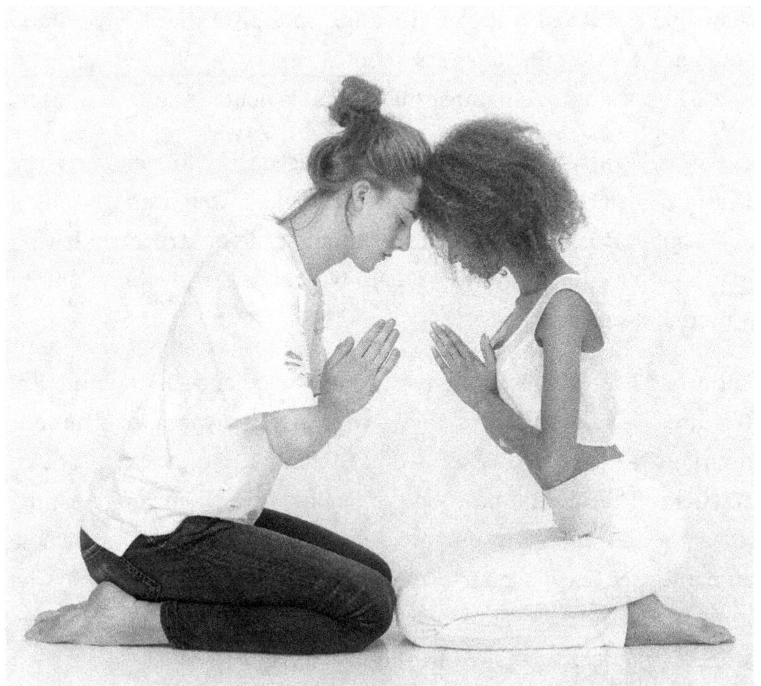

So I didn't go to the original Tantra workshop I signed up for but instead went for my first workshop with Margot. This was way back in the early 1990s.

During that workshop, another dramatic change in my meditation practice happened. I was used to practicing quiet meditation so I would be more connected to the upper chakras, to the air in a sense. I would meditate sitting quietly, doing breathing techniques and feeling a lot of energy. And suddenly, at this meditation workshop, I experienced an active meditation, where everyone's shouting to open all the chakras. My lower chakras opened, I was connected to the earth and then it felt complete. It was a whole different world.

Since then, I have followed Margot and for the last 30 years, I have been meeting her at whatever place she tells me to. She invited me to her first ever teacher training sessions. It was, and it has been, a beautiful time for me!

Tantra is not just about sexuality

I'm a Reiki Master, I teach yoga, and I also perform what we call shamanic practices. However, it is only in Tantra that I have found direct answers, simple answers about sexuality. While this is true, it is also important to remember that Tantra is not only about sexuality.

The word Tantra is from Sanskrit, and according to some experts, Tantra translates to mean weaving. It is like a vision, more than a philosophy. It isn't about adhering to any code or structure. It isn't even a path leading somewhere, because you're already there! Tantra is more like an experience.

And what Tantra is, is using our human experience as the practice. Whether we're meditating, doing yoga or pranayama, or even out running, we practice. When we get together, we practice. You're practicing Tantra right now. You're reading this, when you're eating, when you're walking, when you're using the bathroom...your whole human experience is transformed into the practice. That's why the word "weave" makes sense, because it weaves the human experience into the practice; an ancient way of life or vision.

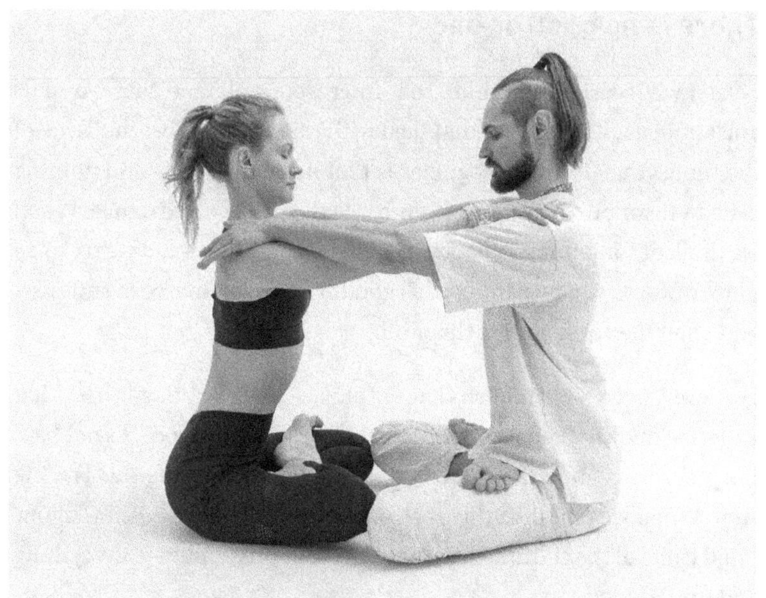

Of course sexuality is also very much a part of the human experience —we all exist because of this energy, we come from it. In Tantra, it is as natural as eating. It isn't forbidden or shrouded in secrecy—it is just a question of channeling this most powerful of energies. And the answers are natural and simple in Tantra.

It is never hard and fast. For instance, in the yogic tradition, there is the concept of Brahmacharya, which people assume to mean celibacy. Charya means path. Brahmacharya literally means the Way of God— the way of Brahma, of the Creator. The way of God is about creation, reproduction. All of existence is the expression of sexual energy. It is just about knowing how to deal with this energy, knowing what to do with it.

Don't waste that energy, but also don't repress it, because then it is just a dormant volcano, a bomb ready to explode. Humans have repressed that energy for so long, it has become weird and it just explodes in many weird ways. Though sexual energy is so vital, our society doesn't teach us how to deal with it. This is the reason it became the main focus of Tantra. However, Tantra is not only about sexuality, but the place where you can dance with your sexuality and embrace it in a natural way.

There is no good or bad

Sexual wellness is something that interests us all, and there are few ancient texts, if any at all, that deal with this. Tantra does, and one of the things that Tantra recognizes is that nothing is good and nothing is bad—it simply causes you to embrace the whole of existence. When we think of something as bad, we want to push it away and we try to go more towards what we think of as good. That is the source of suffering and of all the confusion of the mind.

However, once we establish that nothing is good, nothing is bad, that suffering and confusion retreats. Sexuality... It's not good. It's not bad. It's just reality. It is the same with everything. Grasping this is a big step. When we embrace this realization, it's like a purification of our mind from all the cultural programming. But this applies to everything and to everyone.

Another thing to know about the Tantra vision is that everything is energy, something that physicists are now discovering. Everything consists of energy fields, and matter is like an illusion. The scientists are discovering what the sages have known forever, for thousands of years: that everything is energy. My voice is energy. A table is energy

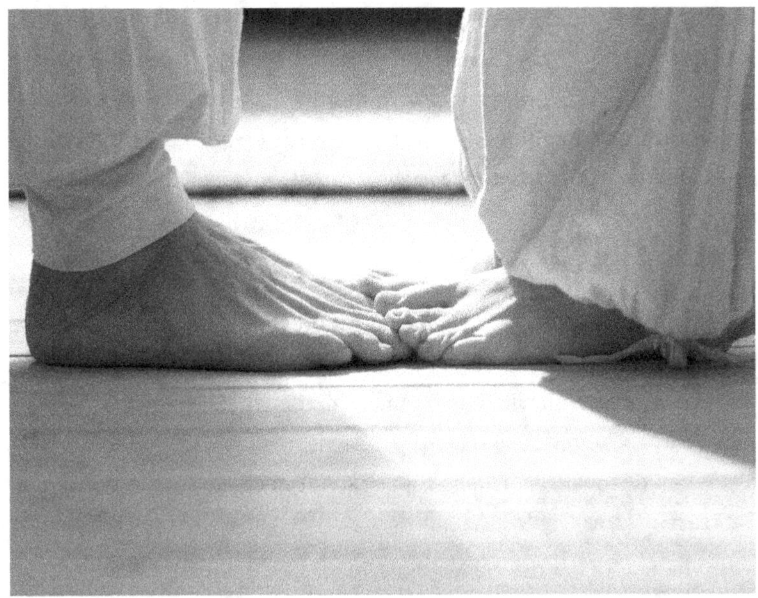

because it's made up of atoms. Sexual desire is also energy that flows through our whole body. The heart is just muscle and it beats with electrical impulses — also energy!

How Tantra works

Tantra helps to understand the energy map of human beings; not unlike other Eastern traditions such as the Chakra system, or the Meridians in Chinese medicine. The energy system is also of great significance in acupuncture and in Reiki, which I have also practiced for many years. The parallels are many.

Tantra also uses visualization; using the miracle of the human mind, the consciousness. We direct energy through our thoughts. For instance, if you start focusing on your right finger, you start feeling your heartbeat there because you're directing all the "prana" there. The prana, or what we call life force in Sanskrit, is used in healing. The yoga nidra techniques use this: techniques of relaxation and self-hypnosis are basically all about visualization. Tantra helps develop visualization techniques to allow us to move the energy. We move it, we embrace it, accept that it is not good, not bad, and that it's all energy.

Now when we see someone and the sexual desire awakens, what do we do with it? We have become accustomed to feeling weird and confused about this desire, which is sad. But what if we embrace that desire, that energy? This is the most powerful energy that we have as human beings. We practice breathing techniques; we guide the energy through visualization. We acquire energy through our breath; our life force. Our visualization guides it, helps us manage it.

Here is an example of how to use a breathing technique: if we take long inhales and then short exhales—it helps charge us with energy. We visualize the heart chakra and we breathe in and out by the heart this way—long inhale, short exhale. Try it! We charge ourselves, we feel the heat and the energy in our hearts. This is also what happens when we make love—using the primal root chakra. We breathe more intensely; we generate more energy. That energy rises and then explodes in an orgasm.

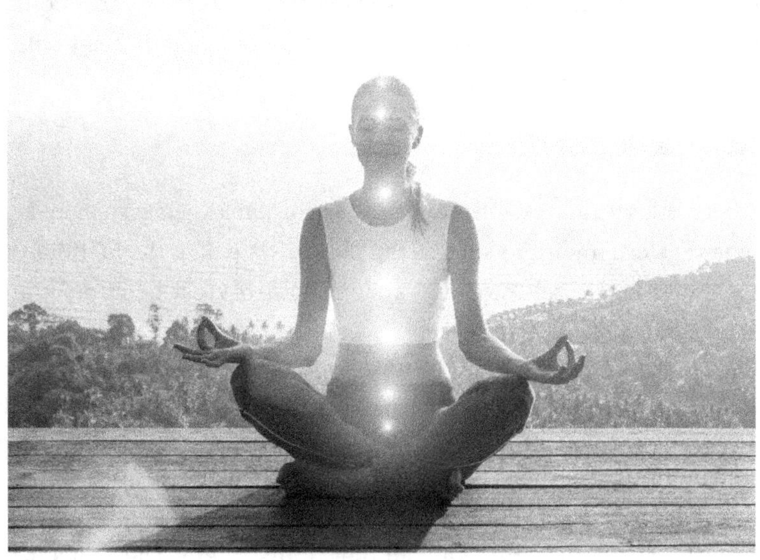

Typically, there is that creeping feeling of guilt right after. We have been conditioned to feel this even when we are with a committed partner. This is why we must try to step into sacred sexuality. We use the breathing technique, we visualize the heart and the color green, which identifies with love. We feel this pressure, we feel the chest opening up, we may start to shake. We are expanding, reaching outward, becoming charged and energized. We feel like we are melting in love, because all of existence is love, it is divine knowledge; just an ocean of love. We become one with everything! You can do this for your sexual partner as well.

You can apply this technique to different situations in life. You can be in a meeting, or your flight was canceled, and you deal with the situation differently. You use Tantra techniques to become compassionate, to slow down your breathing, you direct your energies towards love. You visualize understanding the situation. You can visualize healing as well. Suppose you have a pain in your shoulder, you visualize directing healing energy there via your breath. This kind of healing is seen in a lot of traditions.

Even when eating something delicious, we feel that taste all over, because we're directing energy through the throat chakra to our emotions. We close our eyes to experience the taste all the better. For instance, when drinking wine, we experience with all our senses: vision, smell, taste.

During sex, we breathe into that powerful energy, and we control the experience rather than the experience controlling us. We practice bringing ourselves to this state. We visualize and become aware of the energy. We practice physically as well, by contracting the perineum. For women, it is like holding in the pee; a contraction of the pelvic floor. For men it can be massaging the prostate and other techniques to create sensitivity in the whole sexual area. With practice we are able to isolate the muscles and control each separately to define and refine that experience.

SkyDancing Tantra

Because of the cultural repression around sex, we tend to close ourselves off, but Tantra training is a part of the awakening. We combine all these different strands to create really intense experiences in Tantra. We visualize Shakti and Shiva, the goddess and the god, and we breathe to create a purification process. It's beautiful, and we in the West are only just waking up to it. In recent times there has been a more natural acceptance of sex and sexuality; perhaps there is less repression among younger generations than there was in their parents' generation.

Margot Anand developed SkyDancing Tantra based on ancient traditions as well as modern psychology. Her path of awakening has been helping people reach their potential for 30 years now. It is designed to help people live lives with more love, sensuality and spirituality. Margot is also my teacher and she has been one of the first to teach Tantra in the West. She was a disciple of Osho. I would recommend Margot's books and any Osho writings on Tantra to anyone who wants to understand and clear some concepts. His philosophy is rooted a lot in Tantra.

Margot started teaching Tantra years ago, and because of her background and because she's just this amazing being, she was able to bring this understanding and this knowledge into our western way of life, our way of thinking, our physiology and our mindset. I'm blessed to have been initiated by her; to be able to teach exercises such as this one with the pelvis. In this exercise, you rock your pelvis. While seated, it is a kind of rocking motion where if you push your pelvis forward and backward, you are stimulating that muscle. Margot has created simple exercises like this and certain purification rituals. She guides her students through meditation and visualization; she teaches them how to be able to open and how to love ourselves. We accept that we already are perfect. We don't have to work to be perfect, we don't have to reach some potential. We are perfect *right* now.

Margot brings together these ancient traditions as well as modern psychology. She uses dance to help us. I'm an engineer by training, but then I started to deeply study meditation and breathing. Then I met Margot and started practicing all these different techniques and now my life became my practice. Margot's SkyDancing School, which I think is a beautiful name, is probably the largest and oldest Tantra school in the Western world. I have been studying SkyDancing and I've been training with Margot for 30 years; one among hundreds of teachers around the world.

I have dedicated my life to teaching and sharing what I have learned from my teachers, as the vehicle of my teachers' teachings. I am grateful to my teachers, because they pushed me when I had to be pushed and pulled me when I had to be pulled. It is an honor for me to share with

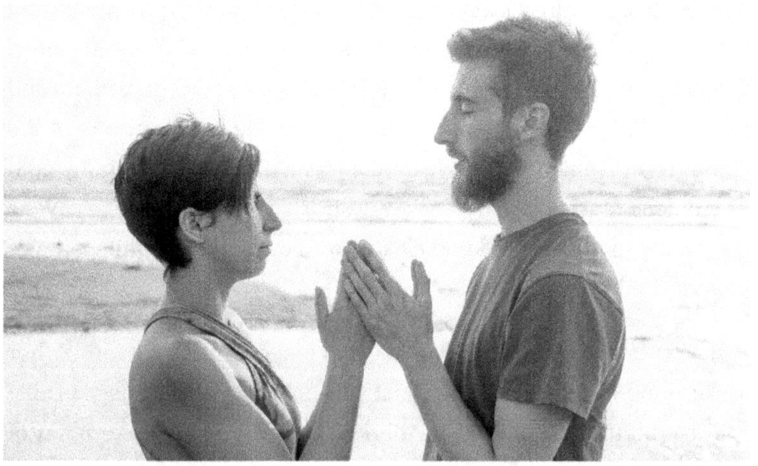

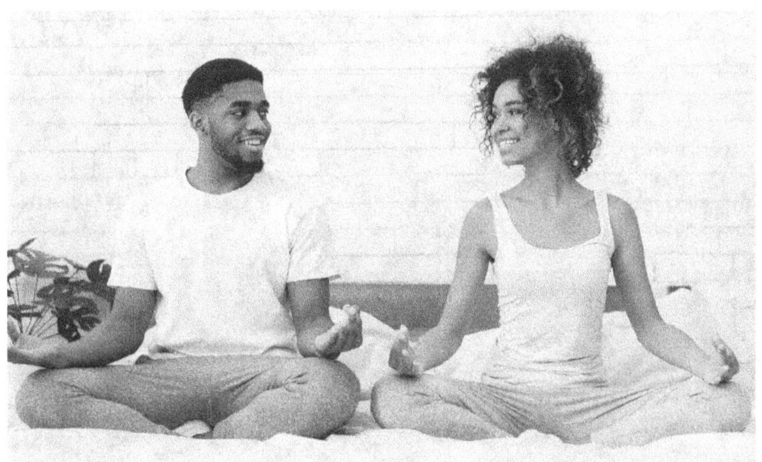

my readers all that I've learned: about my retreats, about tantric spaces, and more. I do two or three retreats each year and I also teach a lot of private classes. I recently moved to Florence, Italy, from where I now conduct my sessions. I do a lot of one-on-one sessions in Mexico City and in New York. I know that I arrive at a place because someone manifested their desire for this to happen. I teach individuals, couples, and small groups.

Students learn the breathing technique with the long inhale and the short exhale; the technique to fully empty the lungs. We learn more about sacred sexuality where we stay in the body and we keep going. We visualize together, and breathe in tandem, in rhythm. We learn to be vibrant, energetic, and healthy.

My teaching sprouts spontaneously, right now I am visualizing doing a training to focus on chakras; so that participants can learn about chakras by feeling them. Exploring the root chakra, which is the source of primal energy, and different types of breathing and visualizations using the "third eye," which is between the two eyes. I hope to continue to help my students the same way my teachers have helped me— to continue along the path of spiritual ecstasy, sexual fulfillment, and joyful health.

The easiest way to contact me is via my email: ulises@yogacare.com or send me a direct message on IG @ulisesyogi.

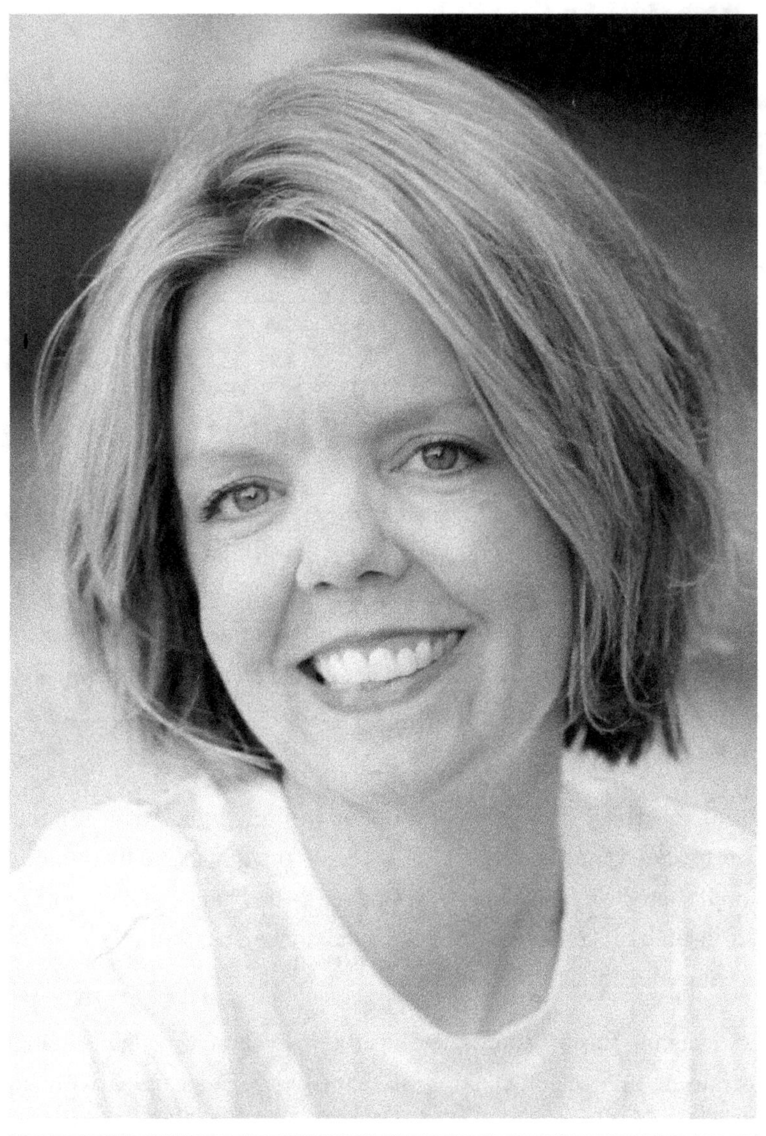

Dr. Kelly Casperson

CHAPTER 7

90% of all urologists are men. Urological treatments have typically centered around the male sexual experience. Hence we find that when women approach a specialist with sexual dysfunction, doctors are often ill-equipped to deal with the situation. Women with sexual health and intimacy issues often have no recourse because medical schools do not fully equip healthcare providers to address these specific female problems. Is it any wonder that we need sex education—adult sex education—for the wider population?

WHY WE NEED SEX EDUCATION FOR ADULTS

By Dr. Kelly Casperson

About three years ago, I had a patient crying in my office because of her lack of sexual function, and I didn't know how to help her. It was a flashbulb moment because I realized something about my medical college training as well as my social conditioning: I was taught that women are difficult, women are challenging, we haven't figured them out yet. I thought to myself, *is it true?* The fact is, we simply don't know, and my medical college training didn't equip me to answer these questions or to treat women such as the one crying in my office either.

Women's bodies are still a 'mystery'

I'm a urologist with a surgical subspecialty. However, we were trained primarily in the male pelvis. We were familiar and comfortable with Viagra and testosterone and the penis and all things male. All the while, I was thinking that other people such as gynecologists were taking care of the women and their sexual health. I later found that I was very much in error there—the gynecologists weren't taking care of the women either!

I started to study this issue and I found that gynecologists aren't taught about female sexual health either. Doctors are taught about avoiding diseases, we are taught about how to not get pregnant—but the average woman and her sexuality and her sexual function? That is just thought of as irrelevant. We are taught nothing about sustaining our sexuality as we age, as our bodies change. We are told nothing about the evolving of a couple's sexual experiences in a monogamous relationship, or how that long duration affects sexuality.

Once I got into this area of work, I was inundated with people coming to me with their sexual health issues. An estimated 40% to 50% of the world suffers from some or other type of sexual dysfunction. This is a staggering number. I realized that there are a lot of people out there who are looking for information, for help. So, I started a podcast three years ago, wrote the book, and did a TED Talk!

Understanding intimacy

Intimacy isn't something we share with everybody. It's something that happens within your personal space, and it's a sign of caring, of loving, of wanting to be near another person. One of the problems is that we've narrowed down sex to fit within the heterosexual paradigm, especially to the penis and vagina. So, if the penis has a problem, or the vagina has a problem, everything stops. People don't realize there are many other ways to be intimate. Even just holding hands can be pleasurable—a form of intimacy.

I was interviewing a sex therapist for my podcast, and I asked, what if a couple hadn't had penetrative sex in a while? Would that be a sexless marriage? The therapist said, we have to back up, and he asked, are they touching each other? Do they even put their hands on each other? This is where we start with intimacy, you can't just jump into penis and vagina sex. Remember, we tried to impeach a president over the definition of sex in the 90s. Is oral sex not sex?

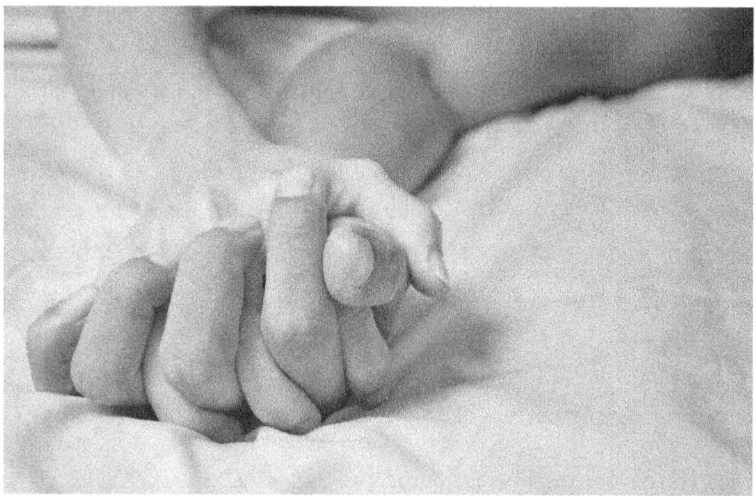

People use different definitions for different purposes, but as far as intimacy and pleasure go, there's a whole cookbook of possibilities that people can miss out on when they interpret sex too narrowly. I was talking to a couple recently and the woman explained how she loved sex before they started having penis and vagina sex. Once they started doing that, it wasn't fun for her anymore because that was *all* that was on the menu then.

The diversity of pleasure can get lost somewhere if we define sex too narrowly. For some couples there is no penis and vagina sex—for them, there's no finish line either. For a lot of women, penetrative sex is actually *not* the preferred method of pleasure. However, there is a lot of ignorance and reluctance surrounding all of the other forms of intimacy. It is also a problem that there is a performative aspect to sex among a lot of couples. A lot of people have some set idea of what sex entails, what it should be, look like, sound like.

There is really a lot of misinformation around sex and at least some of the blame goes to the way it is portrayed in popular culture. Hollywood has had a particular way of showing sex that is rather narrow in its expression. Porn informs a lot of what young people understand about sex; this causes confusion and adds to the problem of misinformation. The repressive ideas propagated by religious taboos and disapproval expressed within some families only further complicate the issue.

The female orgasm

Only an estimated 30% of women are able to orgasm with penetrative sex, and usually even those 30% are getting some sort of clitoral stimulation. However, popular depictions of sex in movies and literature would have us believe otherwise, leading to a lot of women feeling inadequate for not being able to orgasm through penetrative sex. The clitoris is actually central to female sexuality and orgasm. However, it is completely overlooked during sex education, even though the clitoris is the penis homologue. The vagina is not the organ of pleasure but this is simply not a widely enough known fact.

Freud has a lot to answer for in the way that he set up sex. He basically said vaginal orgasms are adult and clitoral orgasms are immature. Back in Freud's day, they actually performed some surgeries to move the clitoris closer to the vagina to try to have "adult" orgasms. This is one example of the mis-education and all the damage done, simply because people had a problem admitting that women achieved pleasure in ways other than putting something in the vagina.

To put it plainly, people simply don't know how women achieve pleasure. Hollywood movies and porn aren't a great way to get an education in sex. Most of the time, people are performing in ways they think they *should* be performing. There is no education that not having a vaginal orgasm is perfectly normal, or that orgasming in a different way is actually far more "normal."

We want to have more sex when we enjoy it. If we don't enjoy it, we have less sex, this leads to low sex drive and then it becomes a self-perpetuating problem. Stereotypically, a man brings the woman to the doctor: she's broken because she doesn't want to have sex. What the man doesn't realize is that simply putting a penis in the vagina is not bringing her to orgasm. He doesn't realize that it is actually really boring for her. She doesn't want to have that sex. Further, there could be issues surrounding vaginal dryness, pain, and discomfort that further complicate the issue, which this perfectly well-meaning man may be oblivious to.

Shaming women for experiencing desire

We've got images of fetuses masturbating in utero, proving that this is a natural, pleasurable activity. The index finger is amazing. So is the vibrator. And yet somehow, society is much more comfortable speaking about male masturbation than female masturbation.

There is a socio-cultural context within which sex exists and we have to see it that way. Historically, female pleasure itself has been seen as problematic. Over the ages, women have been shamed for feeling desire and have been told that their bodies are dirty. Basically women have been kept uneducated about their own bodies, probably as a form of control.

Women are told to guard against pregnancy and therefore refrain from sex. This has been a way to make women fear sex and control them over the ages. Boys and men are socialized to always want sex—this is seen as "normal" and condoned by society. However, women are socialized differently. Women who owned their sexuality have always been seen as misbehaving, as "bad." Society approves of women who restrict sexual activity to happen within a marriage.

We "slut-shame" the women that express desire. However, that same desire becomes acceptable within a marriage—after which she is supposed to desire all the time—in other words, as much as her partner does. This is why the socio-cultural context really matters, as does religion and the learning we receive from our parents and our teachers. Plus, there is Hollywood telling us what desire should look (and sound) like. That's a lot of pressure! In the middle of all this, it is difficult to navigate this world and to figure out what is "'normal." It is difficult to unlearn what is essentially a really bad education.

Relationship vis-à-vis sex

We are also often uninformed of what a relationship can look like, what it *should* look like. A relationship is about intimacy, and being intimate isn't just about the sex. It is about the closeness between two people; it is about the whole picture. It is about thinking, *what does my partner need to really make it an exceptional experience?*

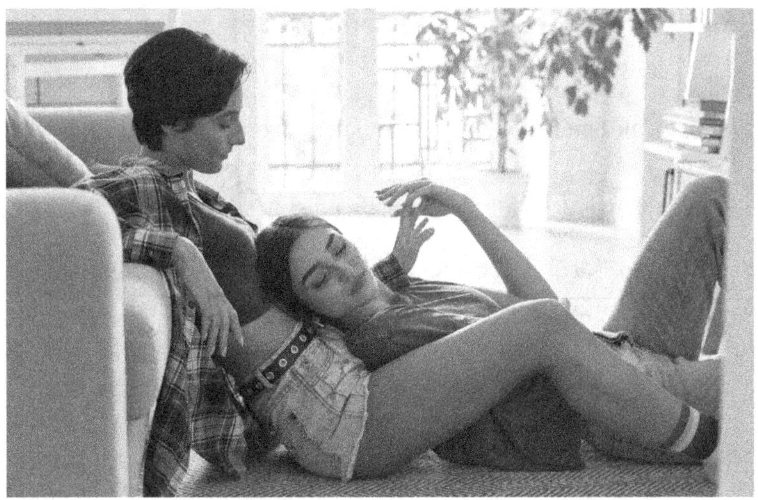

And that's the other thing, it doesn't have to be exceptional all the time, every time. The well-known sex therapist and couples' therapist Barry McCarthy talks a lot about long-term relationships and about making sex work long term. And he has this concept called "good enough sex." This means that some of the time, if the sex is just good enough, that is okay. The idea that it is necessary to experience an orgasm each time is too much pressure. Sometimes it's enough to just be together, to have good enough sex, to keep it going. That's perfectly okay.

Knowledge is empowerment, communication is vital

Information and education are vital. It is how we become empowered. Because women don't *know*, women don't feel empowered, or safe, or healthy to explore their own body. As things are, they put that power in the hands of their male partner.

We see this in the language: he *gives* me an orgasm; he gives me pleasure (or doesn't give me pleasure). How is this even possible when he doesn't even have the same body part? The man certainly does not have any greater education than the woman, because it is she who owns the hardware, so to speak.

This is why communicating with a partner is hugely important. We have to learn to communicate about sex, to explain what feels good and what we like. Talking about the lack of knowledge is important too. Either way, education is empowerment; it is vital for understanding what pleasure feels like in your body.

Communication is an important precursor to connection. Connection, in turn, is vital for relationships. While some people feel connected via sex, some need to feel connected before sex. It is important for a couple to know what makes them feel connected, and so again, communication is the key.

A lot of couples get into routines over time. They might start doing the same thing over and over, and they don't talk about it. It becomes easy to do this—these are known as "sexual scripts." The challenge is firstly to identify and then to break out of that sexual script; to examine if this is all there is. Could there possibly be more? Can we talk about it?

Another communication tip is to communicate afterwards. It can be something simple like: *that was really great.* Or *that was super fun, remind me to do that again.* It is simple—you're just reflecting that it was good. A big part of what makes us feel connected is the intimacy after sex, such as cuddling. This feeling safe afterwards, being held afterwards is important, too. Not knowing that about your partner limits your connection.

Communication is also important for couples later in life—when issues such as vaginal dryness, erectile dysfunction and so on become common. At this point, there is all the more reason for couples to communicate—to express what they like, what feels good right from the beginning. This communication stands them in good stead in their senior years.

Embracing technology

Think about an itch we can't scratch. We typically have no problem asking a partner to scratch, say, the middle of our back because we cannot reach there. We have no problem saying exactly where: a little to the right, a bit higher, etc. Why then do we have a problem giving other kinds of direction?

There is still a stigma around women asking for pleasure. We think about sex as somehow unique in our world, when it really isn't. I have an electric toothbrush, and I use a Waterpik flosser. I've two pieces of electronics to clean my teeth. It is known that they clean teeth better than a manual toothbrush.

We use technology for everything, but we think of sex as unique. We don't associate technology with sex. It is the only area of life where we *think* we are not allowed to use technology; because of what we call sex exceptionalism. Yes to technology, but not in the bedroom.

It is the same with using lubes. The clitoris is not self-lubricating and neither is the penis. Oftentimes the vagina is unable to self-lubricate— arousal non-concordance as we call it—because of age, or surgery, or another reason. There isn't enough lubrication but people are hesitant about using a lube. Why are we relying on just four glands to do the job of lubricating everything! It's just not right.

Studies show people who use lube find it easier to orgasm.[1] Lubrication is great, but I see a lot of resistance around its use. Some women have boyfriends that don't want to use it. Some boyfriends assume that a woman is not turned on because she isn't wet enough. So, it's the man telling a woman what her moisture means and whether she should use lube or not.

In heterosexual sex, many couples start by penetrating with inappropriate arousal of the woman. An erect penis is not enough. A woman's erectile tissue needs to be engorged. The female pelvis has to be aroused sufficiently before accepting something into the vagina. The vagina lengthens and tips to decrease pain, and that's where the lubrication comes from. Just starting by putting an erect penis in the vagina is painful because the woman hasn't had time to create the moisture. And then the man tells her not to use lube and he is setting that woman up for not liking sex.

Female sexual health vis-à-vis male sexual health

As I said before, as a urologist, I was trained to address male pelvic health rather than female pelvic health. Urologists are on the forefront

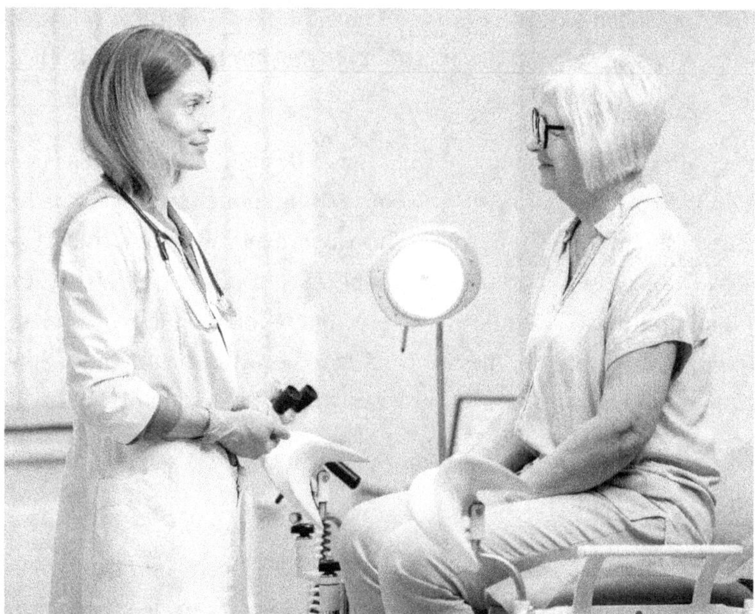

of the Viagra world; doctors write out about a million prescriptions for Viagra a year in the United States. It's one of the most common medications worldwide!

Interestingly, about a million women in America go into menopause each year as well, but most are receiving no treatment. About 4% to 7% of menopausal women get treated for genitourinary syndrome of menopause. Now, if we assume that about 90% of men are heterosexual, and they have this new super penis, did they communicate with their partner? Are they asking: *Hey, am I taking care of you to be able to accept this super penis? Is this even what you want?*

I think urologists and doctors in general, have done a big disservice to people by treating the male and giving him erections, but not treating his partner. And a lot of doctors will say: *I'm just here to take care of the person in the clinic room with me.* However, there's evidence to show that giving Viagra to the man and not treating his partner can actually destabilize a relationship.[2]

Men often have some (often erroneous) ideas of what a woman wants and they will come to me for Viagra. I ask whether they are married and whether this is something their wife wants. Nine times out of ten, the man doesn't know because he hasn't talked about this with his wife. When I ask, *what are you going to do with this new penis*, they don't really know!

Very often, all she wants is for sex to not be painful. Maybe it's been painful for a long time or she just isn't getting enough arousal. Usually, the couple isn't using lube, nor is she using vaginal estrogen to address her menopausal symptoms. The couple may have stopped having sex a long time ago. He thinks it's an erection problem. But her problem was very different! So, they stop going to bed at the same time, they stop holding hands because in a sense both are afraid of what will happen—or rather not happen.

"You Are Not Broken"

You Are Not Broken—Stop "Should-ing" All Over Your Sex Life is the title of my book. This is my way of helping to bridge the gap in healthcare for the women whose confidence is broken, who either don't desire intimacy or desire better intimacy. I have found that the women who meet me in my office are hungry for education and for better sexual health.

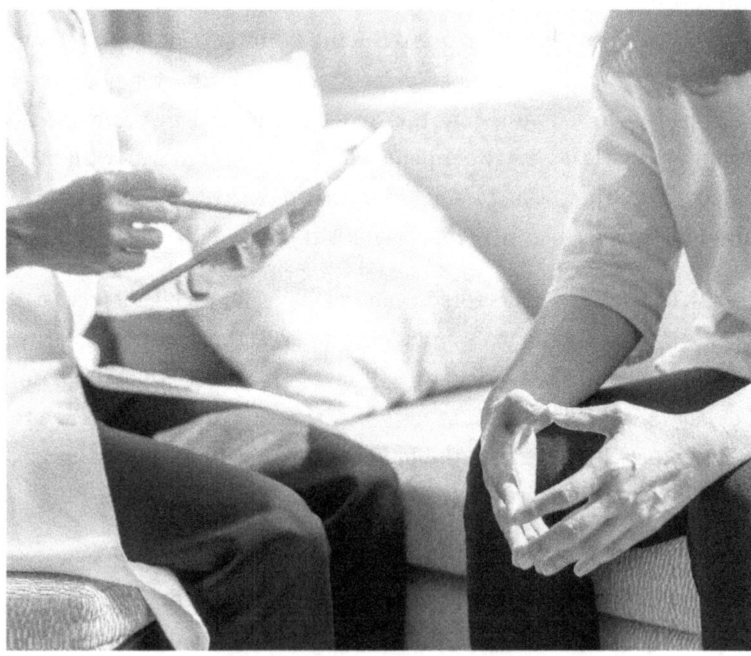

We all need to get over the idea that someone or something is broken. No one is broken. I came across a 74-year-old couple that hadn't had sex in a very long time. They got busy, older, they had knee replacements. Then at age 74, they discovered they both like sex a lot and they're having sex four times a week. I just prescribed some vaginal estrogen and sex is even better now.

It's possible. You have to stay curious and you have to be willing to fail. It isn't a race, nor is it a test we're going to be graded on. It's okay to fail. It's okay to have mediocre sex sometimes. It's okay to be tired sometimes. We put too much pressure on ourselves to be a certain way, and that isn't how it has to be.

My mission is to educate adults about sex. I see them suffer simply because they don't know basic facts and feel really bad about it. They get disconnected from themselves, their own bodies, their pleasure, and their partners.

We have to keep talking—about sex

If I could, I would hand out vaginal estrogen to everyone—and I would continue to talk, because I hope for the message to resonate enough to actually bring about a cultural change. We have to talk about it, normalize it. We have to ask *what do I want*—because the answers can actually lead to personal growth. Effective communication leads to personal growth.

We have to get over the idea of sex being somehow dirty—we made those rules somewhere along the way, and we get to decide to undo those rules. If some cultural rule isn't serving me as an adult in my sexual relationship, then that rule needs to change.

The clitoris is vital but it is a completely ignored organ. It is there for a reason and we shouldn't neglect it. Let's not pick on men for not knowing where it is—they don't have one. It is okay for a woman to show them, to tell them how to touch, to do what gives her pleasure. Again it comes back to communication—and if you find that that needs an adult, sex ed masterclass, well, then educate yourself!

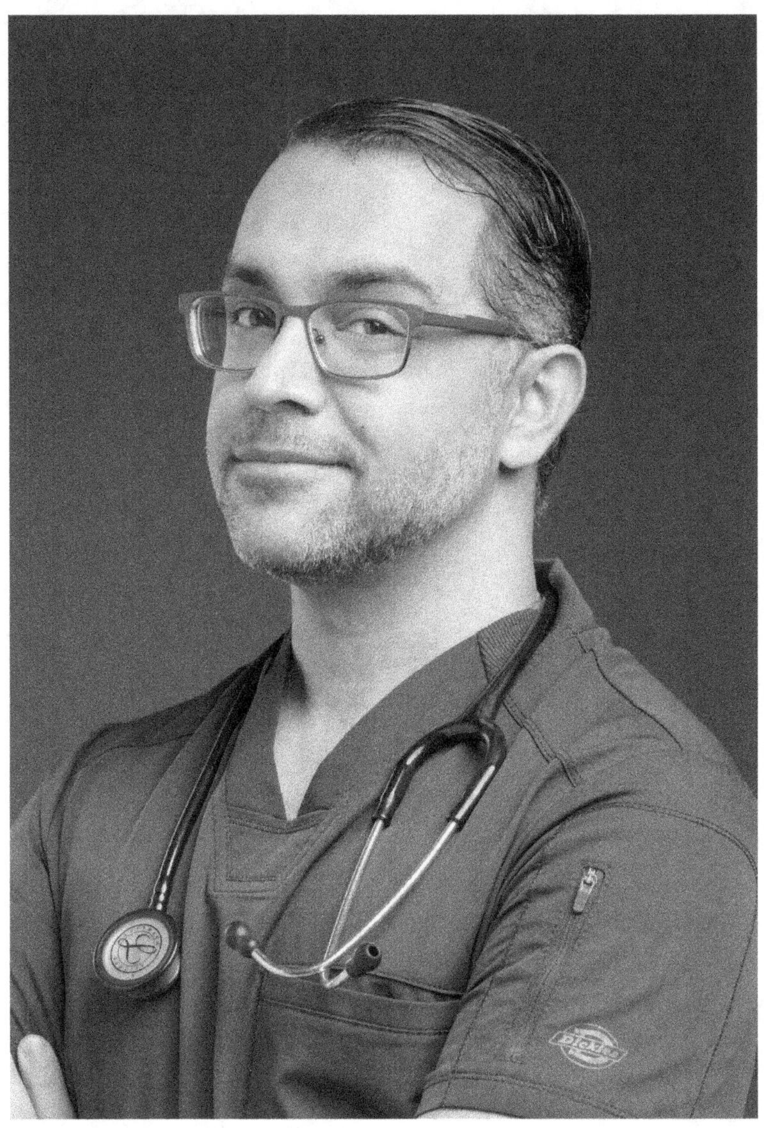

Dr. Siyamak Saleh

CHAPTER 8

A lot of kids today get their sex education from inauthentic sources instead of their schools or their parents. As such, there are a lot of sexual myths that people believe, and there is widespread misinformation that unfortunately is treated as gospel truth. For instance, there are many alarmist posts surrounding masturbation that misguide young people. There are many myths about virginity and the hymen. There are numerous scams and products that claim to help people overcome sexual dysfunction or promise penis enlargement that fool people. There are other sexual myths out there about pregnancy, mental health, and STIs, about sex in the older population, and more. This makes it all the more important to become educated about sex and to communicate clearly with a sexual partner in order to enjoy good sexual health.

HELPING BUST SOME SEX MYTHS & IMPROVE RELATIONSHIPS

By Dr. Siyamak Saleh

I am a medical doctor and a social media influencer with more than three million followers. I have made it my work to bust sex-related myths using TikTok, YouTube, Instagram, and Facebook.

The kind of messages I get via my DMs are interesting, to say the least. *I kissed my boyfriend, my period is delayed—could I be pregnant?* or *My boyfriend uses his fingers on me and my period is delayed—could I be pregnant?* These are 13, 14, 15, and 16-year-olds, not small kids that are asking me these questions. It is sad how little they know and the reasons are not far to seek. For a lot of these kids, speaking about sex is taboo in their families because they belong to traditional cultures.

Many have had no sex education in school. Some are uncomfortable or awkward about the whole issue and find that they are unable to speak to their parents about sex.

There are so many reasons why young people are getting incorrect, incomplete, and just false information about sex. It isn't just kids—even adults believe some of the sexual myths and the misinformation that are common currency all around us. It is important that we all have access to the actual facts, and to accurate, up-to-date information. This is important because good sexual health is actually a human right.

A *Lancet* article speaks about sexual health, human rights, and law,[1] and explains why sexual health is (or ought to be) a human right. There are somatic, emotional, intellectual, and social aspects of sexual health, which is why good sexual health is positively enriching. It can help us enhance our personalities, interpersonal communication, and our experiences of love. Sexual health isn't just about reproduction and sexually-transmitted diseases, but also about well-adjusted, nurturing relationships, and good quality of life.

Sexual health is vitally important for a healthy and fulfilled life. However, the misinformation and secrecy surrounding sex, and the lack of access to sex education, present a significant problem. This is why I have made it my mission to educate people, and dispel misinformation and bust myths surrounding sex.

The power of social media

I am a general practitioner in a primary health care facility, but my real claim to fame is my reach on social media, which started around three years ago at the beginning of the Pandemic. I started to make videos to raise awareness on women's health, on COVID-19 and the HIV epidemic in South Africa. And I was busting myths! In a series of about 10 videos, I put out information to help dispel some of the common misconceptions around sex. These videos went viral and got over 30 million views. With the amount of misinformation out there, I decided to take the responsibility to use my platform to educate people on their sexual and reproductive health.

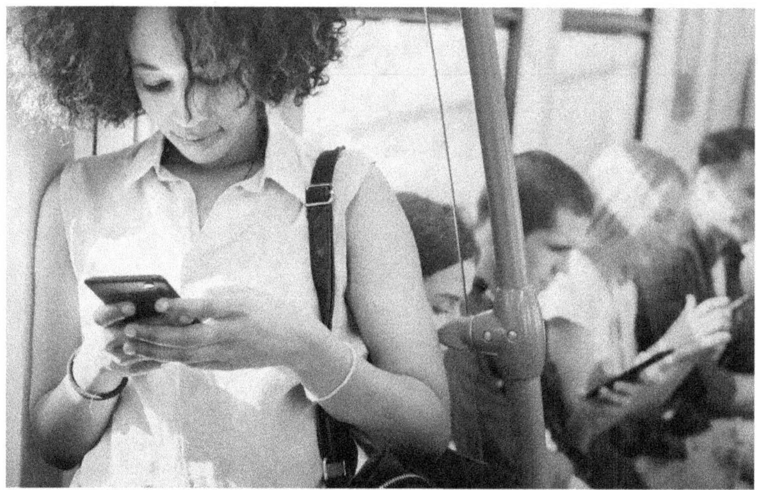

I grew up in the Middle East where we had no sex education to speak of. I learned about sex when I was 14 or 15, and I thought to myself, *that is a lie, my parents don't do these things.* A lot of societies are similar in that there is no sex education and even speaking about sex is taboo. There is no accurate and clear information reaching the kids; just hearsay and distorted, incomplete information from friends and maybe from porn. So how do we resolve this?

While in a lot of western nations, kids are prescribed comprehensive sex education in schools, this is not true for more traditional societies. It is still something that families do not speak about; like some secret to be hidden away. Parents don't talk to their kids about sex because it is awkward and embarrassing. And kids don't really have access to authentic and reliable sources of information. They end up getting half-baked and often completely inaccurate information from friends, porn, and the internet.

I have all sorts of queries in my DMs: *please guess the father of this child,* asks one. *How can I have a twin?* asks another. *How can I conceive a boy?* another wants to know. When I reply by telling them that these questions have no answers, they get upset and want to look for the answer elsewhere. The fact is that there is just so much ignorance and misinformation out there about sex—billions don't yet have access to the human right called sexual health!

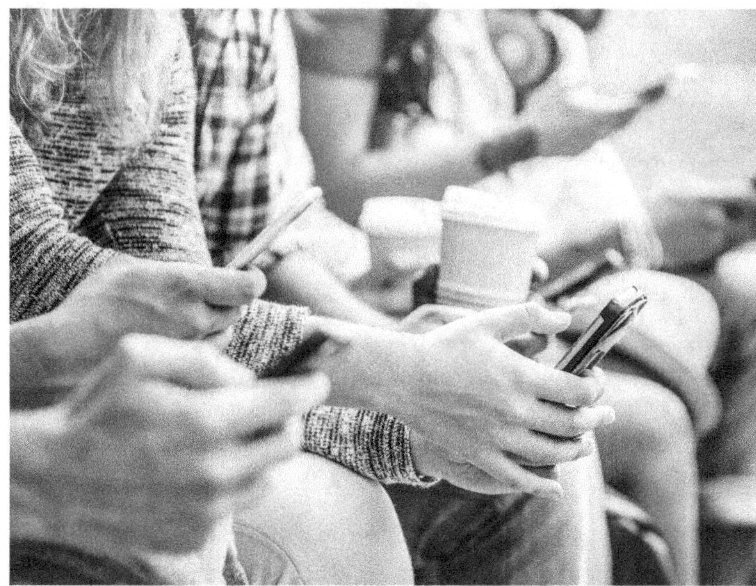

We need to make a lot more effort. Social media is a great tool; a powerful driver for education and information that can reach even the remotest and least privileged communities. People may not sign up to a sexual health presentation for 45 minutes. However, short videos lasting a few seconds or minutes, and succinct, informative posts can be engaging and educative, too. We make it more fun, simpler, and easily digestible. This is information for youngsters to watch and learn effectively and effortlessly.

Busting sexual health myths

One of the most common myths about sex is that a woman cannot get pregnant when she is on her period. This is simply not true and it is easy to see how such an erroneous belief can lead to some very unfortunate consequences. The fact is that the sperm can live for up to five days in the vagina. So among women with short cycles, say a 21-day cycle, ovulation can occur just a few days after their period. Hence, pregnancy can be a very real possibility even if sex only occurred while a woman was on her period.

Then there is the myth surrounding natural lubrication of the vagina. Arousal does not necessarily result in lubrication. So, a lack of natural lubrication cannot be seen as some type of inadequacy or an affront to either partner. Stress, medication, menopause, etc. could mean suboptimal lubrication, but this need not be a problem. A water-based lubricant is a safe, simple, and effective solution. This enhances enjoyment and reduces pain and friction. The use of lubes is not a comment on either person's sexual prowess!

One of the key ingredients of a good sexual relationship is communication: when partners can and do tell each other what works for them honestly and openly. For instance, sex toys may be something one or both may want to try out. These again are no comment on either partner; just the desire to be inventive and/or adventurous.

Another sex myth is the one surrounding aphrodisiacs. Chocolate is supposed to give you better sex, oysters will turn you on, they say. These claims, however, are good only for selling products—for chocolates on Valentine's, and expensive oysters. There is no scientific basis for these claims. There is no proof that chocolate increases your libido or sexual arousal.[3] That said, if the chocolate or the wine or oysters makes one happier and more excited, then maybe there's no reason not to have these food items.

Does size matter?

Another one of the issues I frequently encounter is the anxiety around size and the desire for penis enlargement. One of the biggest myths on social media is it is somehow possible to grow the penis and make it bigger. This is just a scam. If men took the time and energy they waste in this useless pursuit and instead used it to learn some techniques and to get to know their partner's body, this would actually improve their sex life. There are many ways to last longer, to combat aging, such as Kegel exercises, which are beneficial for both men and women. This can help have a better sex life than buying the scam oils and pills that do nothing to change the penis size.

A study examined female preferences regarding penis size and found that women are not overly concerned with penis size—the preferred size is only slightly larger than average.[2] There are far more important criteria than that for women, such as attraction, comfort, emotional attachment, and attractiveness. Penis size comes rather low down on the list of priorities. It is possible to have satisfying sex without a penis in the mix—there are fingers, there is the mouth—the possibilities are myriad.

There is actually a lot we can learn just from YouTube. There is Educational Porn, where the actors stop halfway, and educate viewers on how to do what and why. Sex is not what regular types of porn shows us. It is more important to make the effort to learn skills, to pay attention not just to the physical but also the emotional and psychological aspects of sex.

Masturbation and other myths around male sex

There is a lot of peer pressure surrounding having or not having sex with kids these days. I have kids asking me whether not having sex as a teenager can shorten one's life or make the penis shrink. Similarly, there are some widespread misconceptions about masturbation, that it can make a person blind, cause them to lose hair, and so on.

Of course, this is not true. Masturbation, in fact, can have several beneficial impacts. It feels good, it reduces muscle tension and mental stress, and can help one sleep better—particularly those who do not have an active sex life. The point is that so long as one is not addicted to masturbation, so long as it does not interrupt daily activities, it is healthy and safe. Sex and masturbation are good for our physical and emotional health. However, addiction or constant preoccupation with sex is not—a distinction to watch out for.

And that brings me to another sex myth—that men think about sex every seven seconds. I did the math and this would mean that men are supposed to be thinking about sex a few thousand times a day! This is clearly not true. In fact, this sex myth is so widely prevalent that they had to do a study to debunk it.[4] Turns out that men aren't nearly as obsessed with sex. The study found that young men think about it about 19 times a day (and women about 10 times a day), but then they also think about food 18 times a day and sleep 11 times a day.

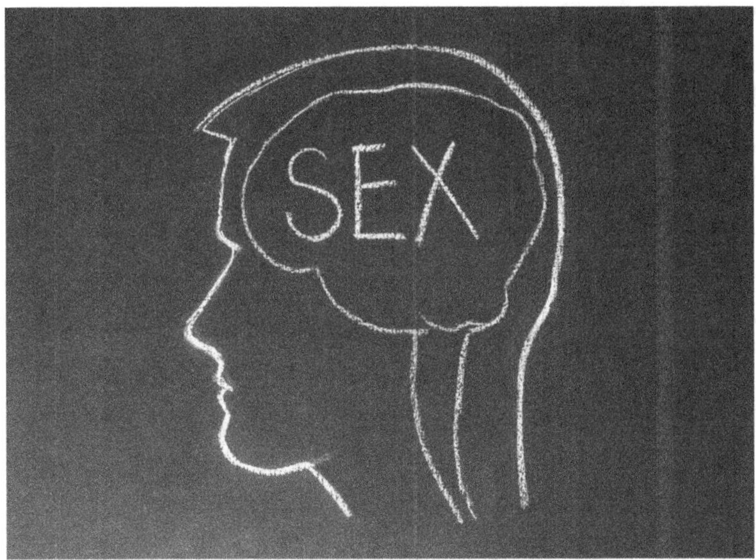

And then there is that story about semen retention—that having sex or masturbating depletes a man. We have athletes not having sex before a game because this will supposedly impact their performance. Again, there is no evidence to back this up. In fact, there could be something to the argument that sex relaxes a person and helps them sleep better —this could end up *improving* their performance the following day!

Myths around virginity and the vagina

There are a lot of myths around the female orgasm. Most women actually do not orgasm during intercourse, and about 75% will need some form of clitoral stimulation to reach orgasm. It is important for women to explore their bodies and identify their erogenous zones. They should pay attention to what helps them reach orgasm, maybe even experiment with a sex toy.

It is interesting to note that all other male and female sex organs have some or other function but the clitoris is made *only* for pleasure. It is also a fact that it has more nerve endings than the penis. However, this organ is still shrouded in a lot of misinformation and mystery.

And then, there is male and female arousal—men are supposed to be quick to be turned on whereas women take longer—is the popular belief. However, this difference isn't as significant as it is made out to be. Psychology plays a role. If a woman is uncomfortable, if she has emotional health issues, all these things will affect arousal and in turn affect her lubrication. It isn't so much a gendered difference as it is an individual difference: it's different for *everyone*.

Foreplay is vital for arousal—the holding, touching, caressing, kissing —there are literally a hundred things that can help to enhance the sexual act. Not only do women find it more pleasurable, but men with issues like erectile dysfunction or premature ejaculation can also benefit.

Talking about women's pleasure, one of the big sex myths is about the impact of sex on the vagina. Some people believe that having a lot of sex will make the vagina lose its tightness and elasticity. This is completely untrue. The only thing that impacts the vagina is childbirth and age.

Patriarchal societies set a lot of store by the "purity" of women's bodies, and by extension, on virginity. Another widespread sex myth is that virginity is something physical, whereas it is more of a cultural construct. In fact, a lot of females are actually born without a hymen.

Some cultures expect women to be virgins on their wedding night and also demand proof of this in some form or other. There is literally no real way to prove or disprove this. In spite of this, there exist surgeries such as vaginal tightening and hymen reconstruction. There are people that will visit a doctor's office to confirm whether or not a woman is a virgin. This is because there is so much stigma around women's bodies and sexuality—which I hope to help dispel.

Sex and weight loss? Maybe not.

This is yet another myth that has gained currency over time—that sex is exercise and that it helps burn calories and aids weight loss. This also has something to do with machismo and the way that men are encouraged to boast about their sexual prowess in a lot of societies.

While sex can burn *some* calories, this is nowhere close to the number of calories required to be burned for weight loss. Some people are upset when I debunk that myth, but then I tell them—carry on, just don't rely on sex as the *only* way to lose weight.

Sex in the later years

A friend recently told me about an amusing and interesting anecdote: the medical clinics around retirement facilities have an unusually high number of STI complaints. Clearly, older people are still having a lot of sex. This busts the myth that sex is for the young. This is notwithstanding the fact that older people more commonly experience issues like vaginal dryness, erectile dysfunction, prostate issues, and so on.

Studies have shown that sex is important later in life as well.[5] About 65% of people in the 65 to 80 years age group said that sex is an important determinant of quality of life. While sexual activity does decline with age, as many as 46% of the age group between 65 and 70 reported being sexually active. As life expectancy continues to increase and quality of life in the later years also improves, sex in the later years becomes all the more important because of how it enhances happiness, health, and well-being. In fact, sex in later years can have a new, relaxed quality to it, since it occurs at a time when people may be retired, have less stress, and have fewer demands on their time.

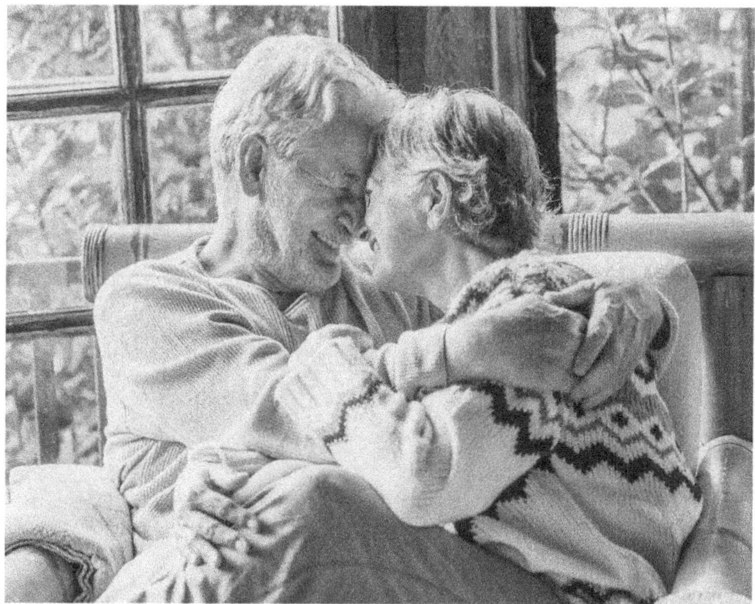

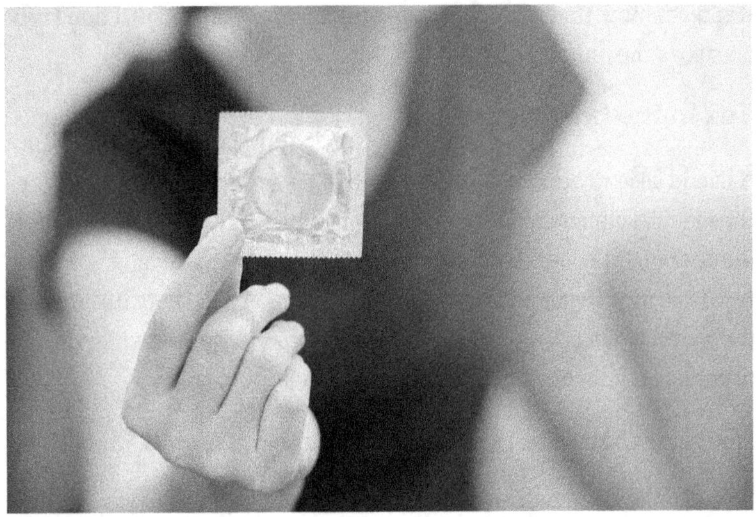

Having a better sex life

To have a better sex life, you need to have a better relationship, as I explain to my social media followers. This is true for any intimate relationship, at any age. Communication with one's partner is vital, and if things are not going well, there is no shame in consulting an expert such as a sexologist. Honest and direct communication not only helps a couple enjoy a better sex life, but it also improves the quality of their overall relationship as well.

Good grooming, looking after fitness, and using some perfume can help enhance one's self-confidence as well as sexual attractiveness. It helps to let your partner know that you're making an effort and that their opinion makes a difference to you.

Educate yourself and become more aware of sexual function and sexual health. If something seems off, don't disregard it. Instead, get help and try to resolve it. Consulting a sexologist, gynecologist or neurologist can be a great way not only to resolve sexual dysfunction, but also to improve one's health overall.

Practicing safe sex is another vitally important aspect of sexual health, regardless of one's age and health status. Contraception is not the only reason to use condoms. As the anecdote about the high rates of STIs among people in retirement communities indicates, sexually transmitted diseases can occur at any age and are important to guard against at all times.

Technology is moving at a fast pace and we will soon have access to the kind of condoms that will be so thin as to be almost imperceptible while still offering protection. Regular screening is another way to avoid STIs—particularly if you are at higher risk of something in particular.

Sex education on social media

What are the factors affecting your mental health? What are the symptoms of breast cancer to watch out for, and is there any way to reduce your risk of this type of cancer? Is period blood dirty like they say it is? Is drinking cranberry juice able to cure UTIs or urinary tract infections? What is the average penis size? Does the morning-after pill impact future fertility? Are AIDS and HIV the same? What are the common causes of painful sex? Is severe period pain just something women must live with? This is a sample of the type of questions I answer on my social media pages.

Via my social media accounts on TikTok, Instagram, Facebook, and YouTube, I work towards empowering people and their sexual health. I try to help improve their confidence and enhance positive relationships, and I hope this chapter has helped you as well.

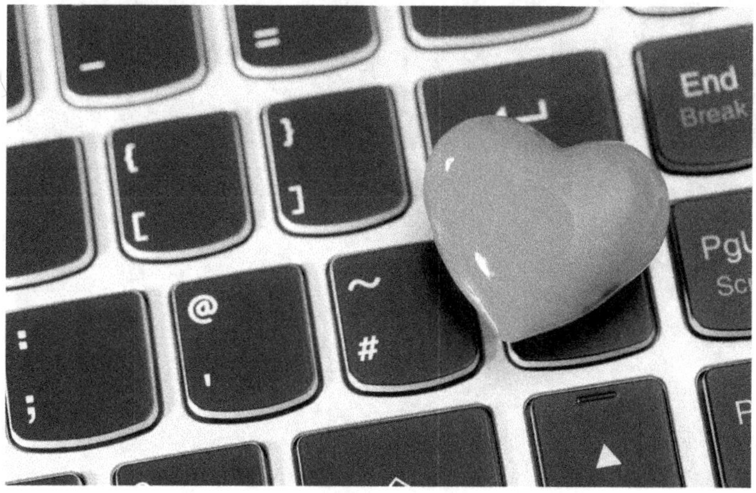

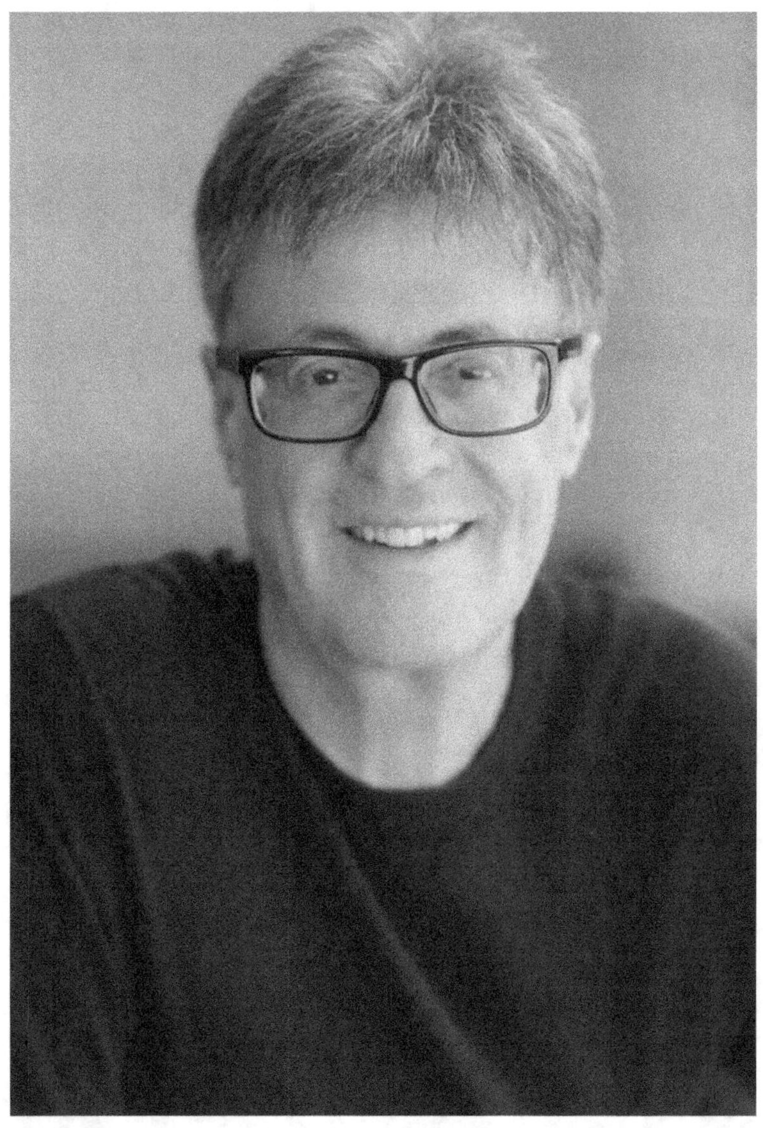

Adiel Gorel

CHAPTER 9

IN CLOSING

By Adiel Gorel

As a person with a life-long interest in health and wellness, sexual wellness is naturally one of the subjects I am interested in. Our sexual energy can be used for healing, enjoyment, and even spiritual growth.

In addition to the Tantra workshops I took with Mantak Chia and Charles Muir, I have done a fair amount of reading into this powerful, yet somewhat under-the-surface energy we possess.

There are various yoga practices that focus on the "feminine goddess energy," and allowing us to learn how to unlock it to enhance our entire body and energetic system, thereby enhancing our vitality and awareness. Terms like "Kundalini" and "Tantra" are common in the space, and volumes are available to read, and learn, in addition to practice.

I was inspired to start my podcast *The Adiel Gorel Show*, after the Public Television show I created called "Life 201." The show is still running as this book is being written.

The podcast involves inviting guest experts in fields I am passionate about, and which I thought would be of benefit to our viewers and listeners. It was an opportunity for me to learn more about the experts' fields, and my "high-tech" mind strove to simplify every expert's message into a form that would be as simple and understandable as possible while offering tangible, actionable items for us to do right now. The podcast allows me to interview these great experts, many of whom have dedicated their lives to a subject that could have great beneficial effects for us. It gives me the opportunity to ask them questions, and hopefully, those Q&As are useful to a number of other people.

Continuing with the "Life 201" theme, we are holding summits on key issues. We had the wonderful Life 201 Breathing Summit, which led to a book called *Life201 BREATHE: Your Path to Improved Wellness Is Only a Breath Away*.

This book is the result of our Sexual Wellness Summit.

As I mentioned, I find the experts who wrote the chapters inspiring and extremely useful, and I try hard as I interview them to bring their knowledge down to earth, as well as find the most useful things we can do in our daily lives to improve our health, with little expense or time commitment.

Every expert who wrote a chapter in this book inspired me and it is my great hope that they have inspired you.

Dr. Felice Gersh talks about how being disassociated from nature is unhealthy in general, and is not healthy for optimal sexual function in particular. She discusses hormonal needs in both men and women. Dr. Gersh explains that "the pill" causes certain disruptions for women, which can actually affect their choice of mate. She explains the natural cycle, and how hormone levels change at different points in the cycle. She explains how men's optimal erections need a low inflammatory environment in the man's body, and how testosterone levels, while generally declining with age, can be higher in healthy living 60-year-olds than in some 30-year-olds. Dr. Gersh highlights the importance of nitric oxide, which was covered extensively in our *Life 201 Breathe* book.

Regarding menopause, Dr. Gersh explains some of the changes that women experience and is an advocate of using bio-identical hormones to mitigate some of the effects. Overall, Dr. Gersh equates healthy sex with a healthy life.

Navin Ramachandran, former COO of the Match Group, and owner of many online dating websites, tells us about his observations about online dating behaviors.

Navin talks about the persistent feeling that someone better is just around the corner, and its effects on the willingness to commit that many people experience in the online space. He talks about how more is less with respect to too many choices. Navin tells us that there are many user profiles still existing of people who are no longer members of a dating website. In addition, he reminds us of the many fake user profiles, and how things may not be what they seem. He talks about different behaviors of men and women, and also LGBTQ+ audiences. He discusses algorithms that dating websites use to maximize profit.

Dr. Vicki Matthews teaches us about the Five Elements. At its core, the Five Elements model is used to describe phases and interactions found in the natural world. The phases are represented by Water, Wood, Fire, Earth, and Metal and can be used to describe anything in the world, including people. Actually, they are especially useful when describing people. Dr. Matthews discusses the nature of each one of these elements, and how we, as people, manifest certain traits and affinities based on our dominant elements. She explains how, in a relationship, it is very helpful to know which elements are dominant in each person and how to harmoniously navigate the differences.

Margot Anand, a pioneer in the tantric field, who is best known for her book *The Art of Sexual Ecstasy*, explains the spiritual aspects of Tantra. She also talks in more specific ways about male and female

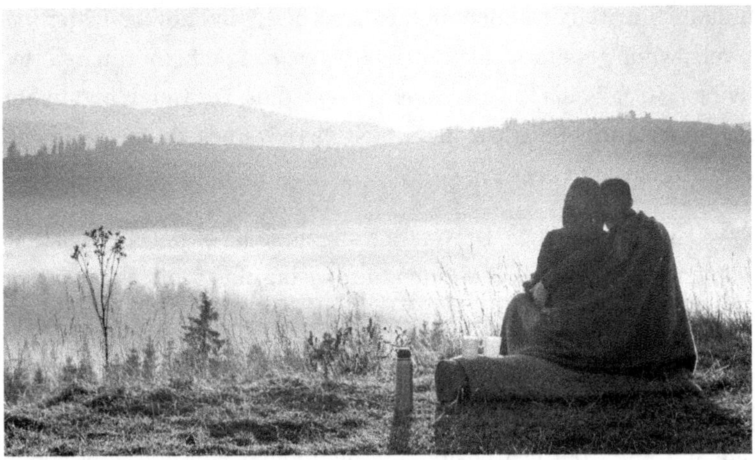

sexuality and orgasms. She talks about "running energy" through our chakras, and gives a specific move we can practice. Margot talks about the art of being "desireless at the height of desire" as a way of being fully in the present and freeing ourselves from the shackles of ego and illusion. And she leads us to reference materials that can further these teachings.

Ulises Calatayud is a tantric master, as well as a Dharma Yoga and Reiki teacher, among other things. He had initially studied with Margo Anand. He talks about harnessing sexual energy for health and spiritual development, with some tangible examples. Ulises explains that Tantra is not just about sexuality, and, in fact, has to do with every aspect of human life. Tantra, in addition to breathing and other energy movement modalities, also uses visualization—using the miracle of the human mind, the consciousness. We direct energy through our thoughts. Thus when we work with breathing or sexual energy, we can direct it via our thoughts to certain parts of the body (or outside the body) for the purposes of healing and development.

Dr. Kelly Casperson discusses the need for adult sex education. She talks about the lack of communication, even in long-term relationships, about sex. She marvels at how many people are afraid to simply share what makes them feel good, so their partner can do it consistently. She talks about people feeling threatened by artificial lubrication, sometimes from an ego place of "I don't need external lubrication. I lubricate enough myself." She discusses the lack of foreplay, of "after-play" and its importance to the connection and to sex. She talks about the excessive weight given to the notion that "sex is only between a penis and a vagina" in heterosexual sex. Kelly talks about actually refraining from "penis and vagina" sex for a while, so as to learn other methods of pleasure and intimacy. She talks about the lack of balance in older age groups, with men who use Viagra pairing up with women who may experience pain and dryness, and how the two don't match. Overall, it is clear that adult sex-ed would benefit most people.

Dr. Siyamek Saleh debunks many common myths in the realm of sexuality. He discusses myths such as: "A woman can't get pregnant while on her period", "Men think about sex every seven seconds", "If a woman is aroused, she won't need lubricants", "sex is better when we are younger", and "size matters", among others. By debunking common myths about issues related to sex and sexuality, he paves a useful road for people to be freed of misconception and enjoy more anxiety-free sexuality.

We hope you enjoyed reading this book, and that you learned a few exciting things to improve your over all sexual wellness and, as a result, your health and happiness.

ABOUT THE AUTHORS

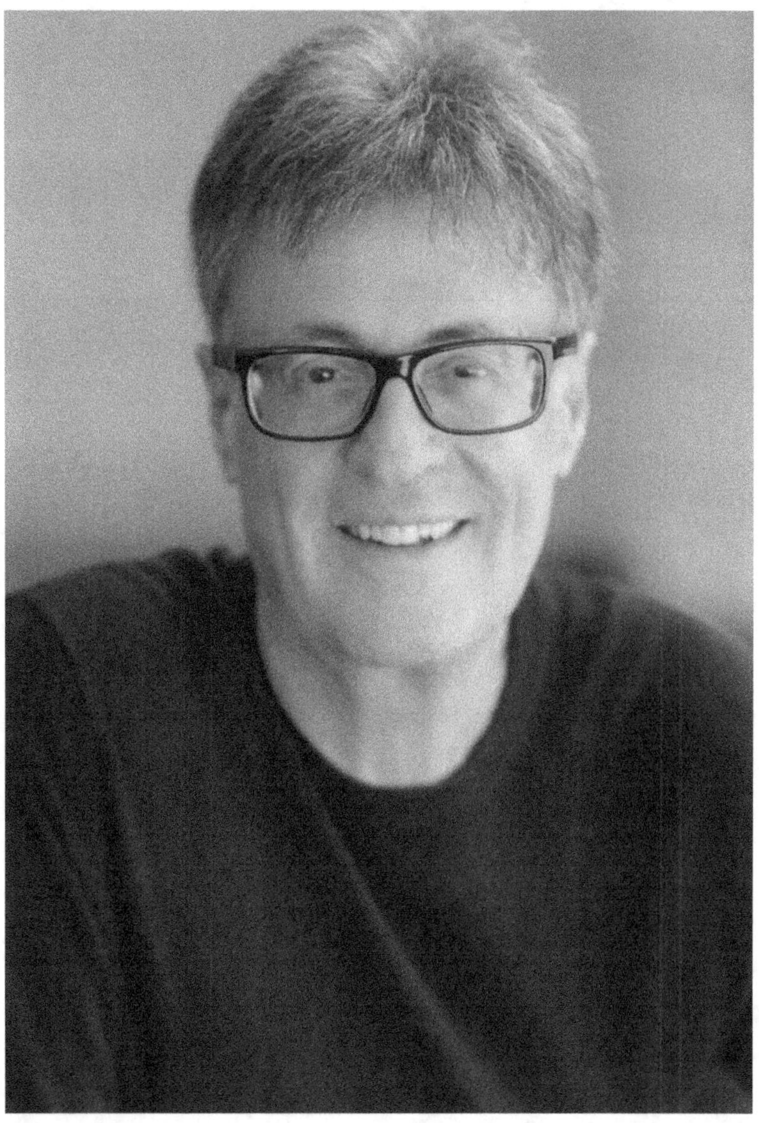

Adiel Gorel

Adiel Gorel

Adiel Gorel is the CEO of a San Francisco Bay Area real estate investment firm and has helped thousands achieve their long-term financial goals. Adiel wears many hats, one of which is that of a passionate health seeker looking to bring about positive change using natural, intuitive methods. Adiel has always been fascinated by the idea of improving every facet of our health, and sexual wellness is an integral part of overall health. Over the years he has read various books, studied the methods used by different sexual wellness experts, and been an avid student of the subject. *The Adiel Gorel Show* is one of the ways in which he strives to get out the message of sexual wellness to his listeners, hoping to drive change via simple lifestyle changes. This book is a labor of love—a collection of essays by sexual wellness experts; people from different walks of life who share their experiences, techniques, and unique insights into teaching us about attaining a healthy sexual life.

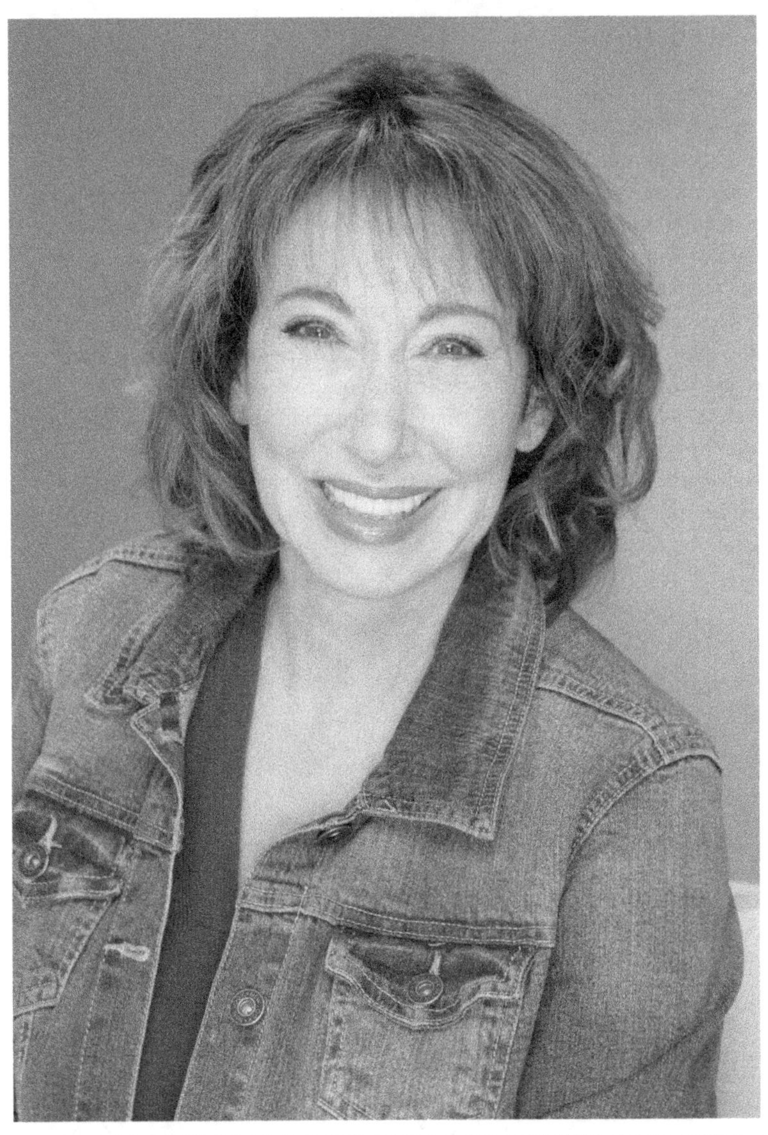

Dr. Felice Gersh

Dr. Felice Gersh

Dr. Felice Gersh is a board-certified OB-GYN and Integrative Medicine physician who applies her dual training and insights to treating and managing complex diseases. She focuses on female health, particularly in the area of hormone management, with a specialization in PCOS. She works in the areas of menopausal transitions, healthy aging, fertility and preconception care, integrative gynecology, and more. Dr. Gersh has one of the most successful private practices in the Orange County area, is a published author, and is frequently called on to speak at international events. She has served on the facilities of the University of Southern California and University of Arizona medical schools, co-authored multiple papers for prestigious peer-reviewed medical journals, serves as a forensic expert, and has won numerous awards for her work.

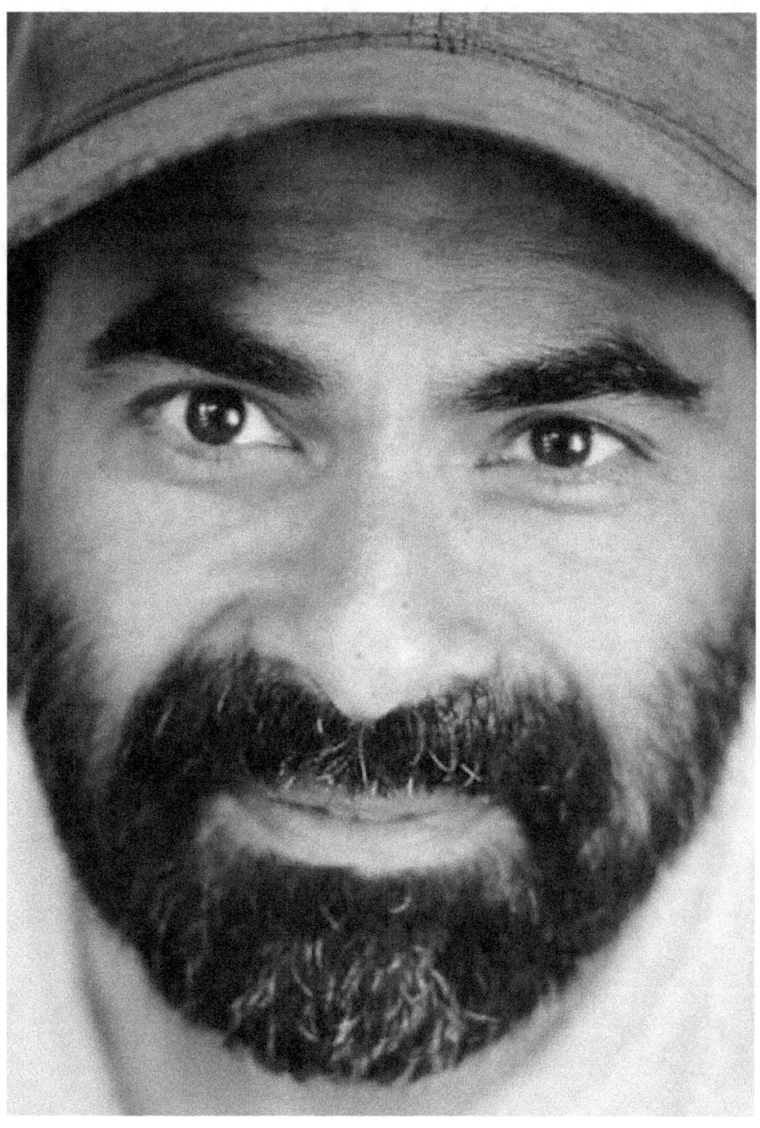

Navin Ramachandran

Navin Ramachandran

Navin Ramachandran was the Chief Operating Officer of Match Group and CEO of Latin America and Asia. He has served in multiple roles within the group as GM of Match Events and GM of Match Latin America. Navin is also an investor and the founder of Gather6, a platform that connects small groups of people through intimate, small-group conversations. He studied engineering in India and later obtained a master's degree in Engineering from Case Western Reserve University.

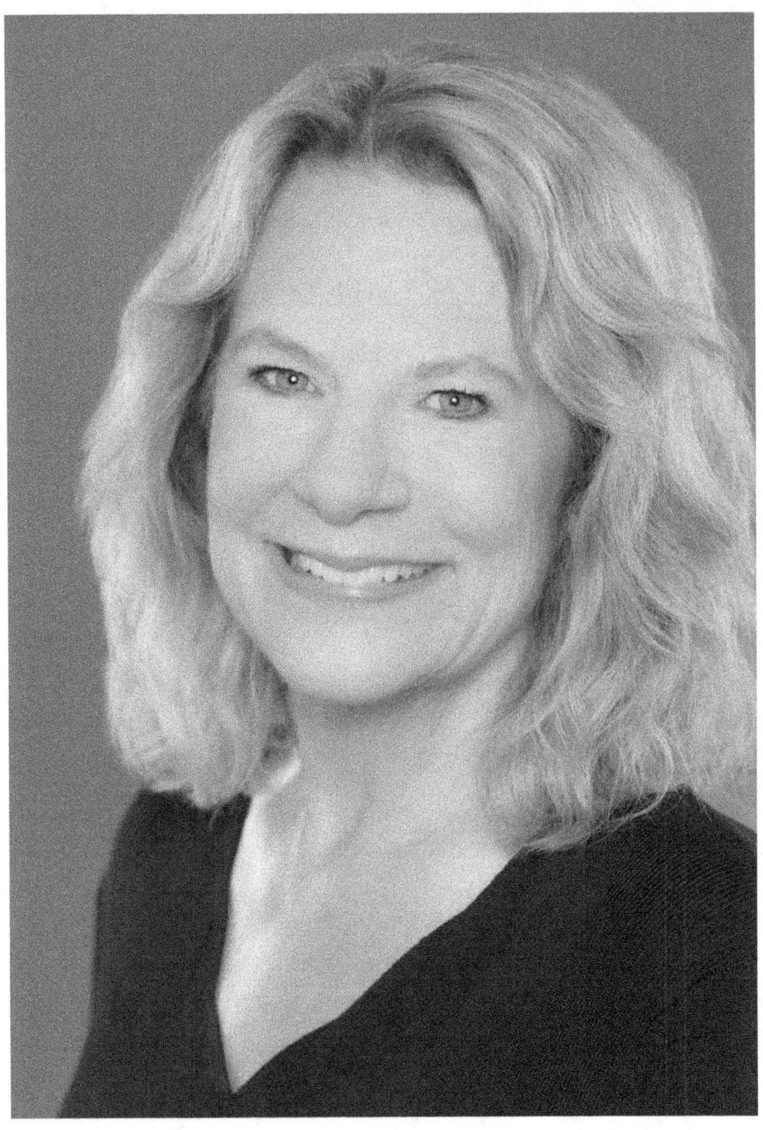

Dr. Vicki Matthews

Dr. Vicki Matthews

Dr. Vicki Matthews is an author, teacher, relationship coach, and naturopathic physician. She is a vocal advocate for natural healing modalities and also holds a bachelor's degree in psychology and an MBA in Consumer Behavior. She has been on the *Oprah Show* twice, and is the author of *The Goddess Letters*, an award-winning novel about the cultural imbalances in the world. Her recent best-selling book, *The Five Elements of Relationships: How to Get Along with Anyone, Anytime, Anyplace*, helps readers improve family dynamics and includes numerous techniques to help build harmonious relationships with everyone. Her Five Elements of Relationships coaching program has helped thousands of people improve their lives and relationships. Information about her programs, books, blog, and speaking engagements are available at: drvickimatthews.com

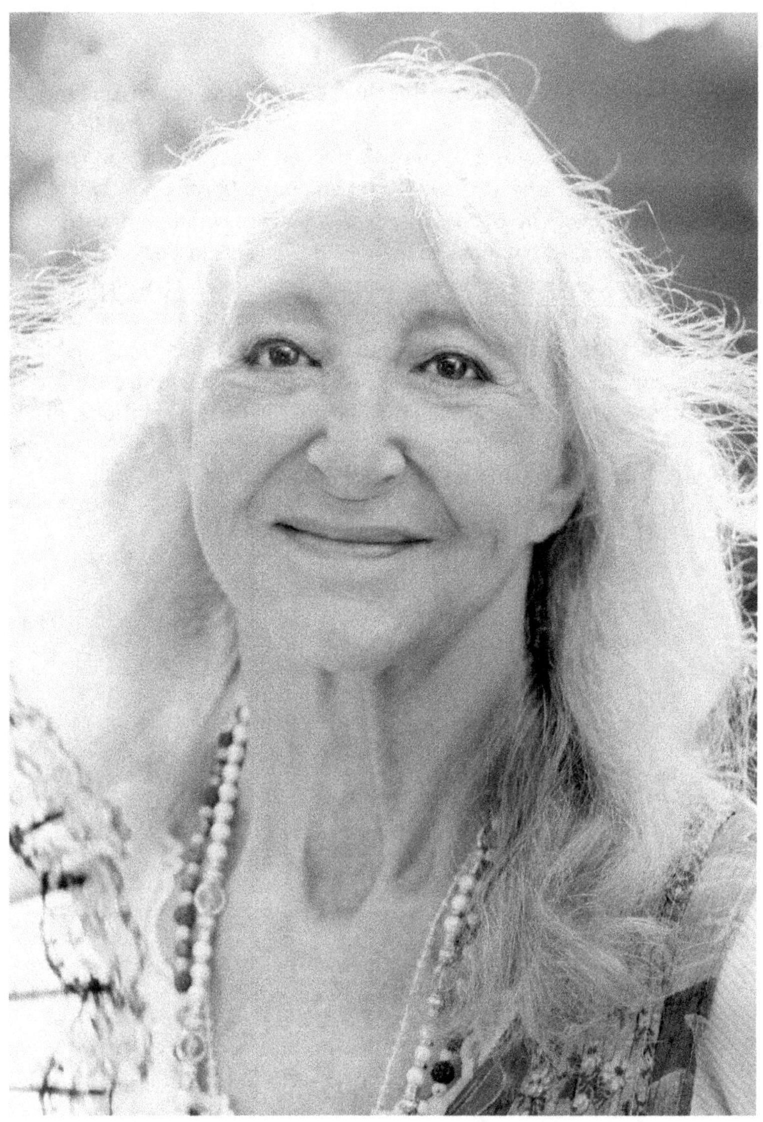

Margot Anand

Margot Anand

Margot Anand is a leading expert on Tantra, and is the author of books such as *The Art of Sexual Ecstasy; The Art of Everyday Ecstasy; The Art of Sexual Magic; Love, Sex and Awakening*, and many more. She started out writing about American pop culture, and then studied Tantra in India in the 1970s under the tutelage of Osho Rajneesh and other masters. Margot Anand was one of the first to introduce the concepts of Tantra and Neotantra to the West. As a much sought-after speaker, she has participated in seminars alongside Deepak Chopra, and taught at Dean Ornish's annual retreats for heart patients. Her SkyDancing Tantra course draws on sexology, music, yoga, and other disciplines. SpiritWorks is her online course that helps cultivate sacred relationships, sensual power, and emotional vitality.

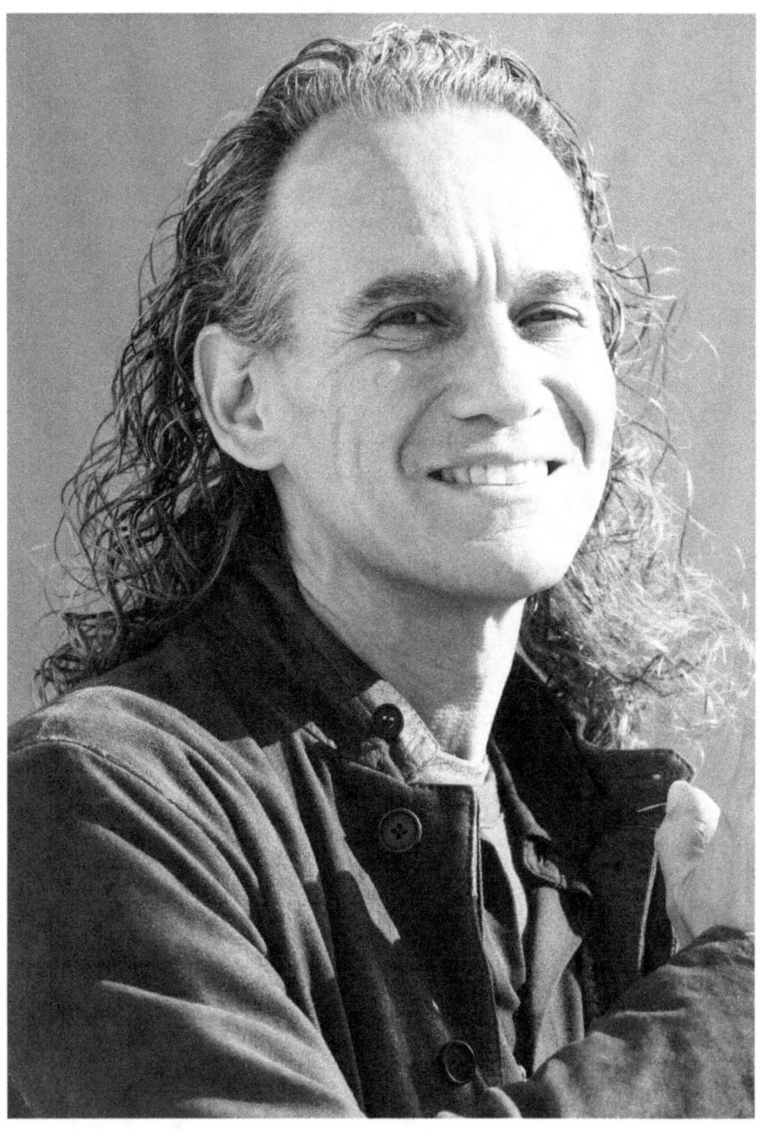

Ulises Calatayud

Ulises Calatayud

Ulises Calatayud is a certified Dharma Yoga teacher, and a
Tantra teacher. Until recently, he worked out of his New York City
studio. He enjoys helping people become the best versions
of themselves. Starting out in the corporate world, he started
to consciously search for that spark that would help light up life.
He has been studying and practicing Tantra, meditation, yoga, Reiki,
and other native traditions for 30 years, and has been teaching
Bikram yoga, breathing techniques, mental physics, and Tantra for
over 25 years. In 2019, Ulises was elected the President of the
International Yoga Sports Federation (IYSF), and has been associated
with Margot Anand for about 30 years. It is his endeavor to help people
integrate simple, natural practices into their lives to achieve peace
and harmony, and to be healthy, youthful and loving.

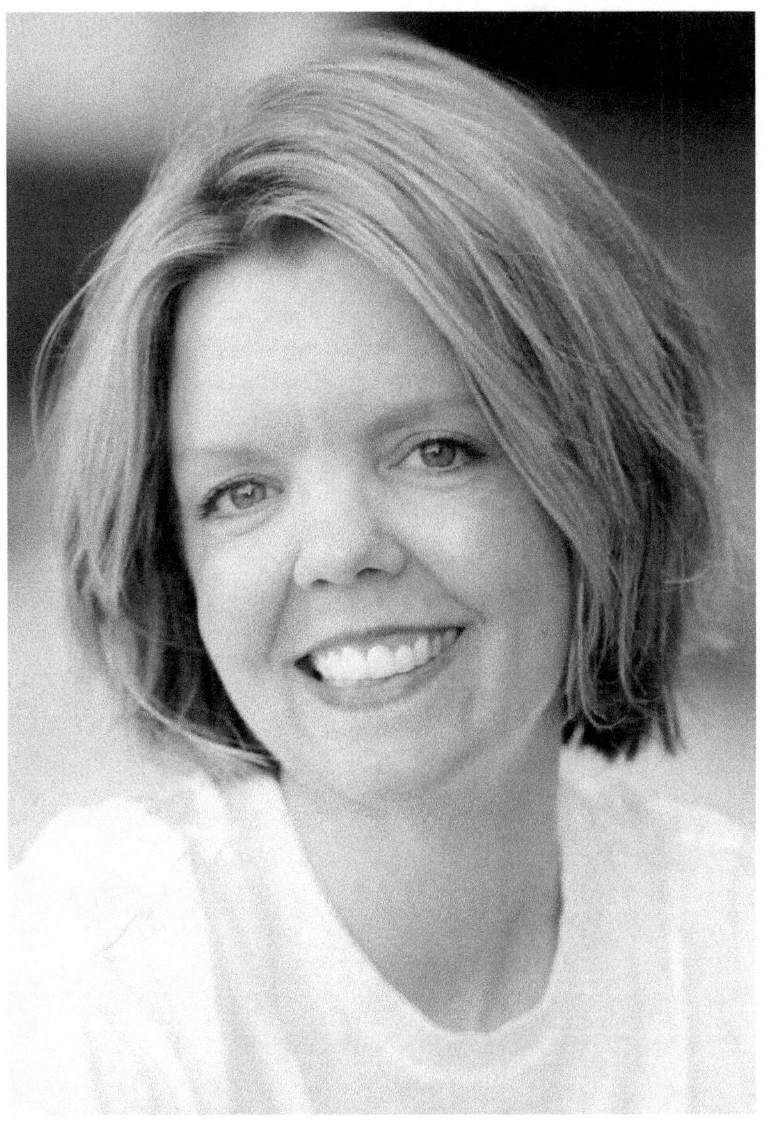

Dr. Kelly Casperson

Dr. Kelly Casperson

"Who is taking care of our (adult) sex education?" asks Dr. Kelly Casperson. Dr. Casperson is a urologist, surgeon, entrepreneur, and educator in female pelvic health. She frequently speaks on sexual wellness, female pelvic health, genitourinary symptoms of menopause, and is an expert in female urology or "urogynecology." It is her mission to empower women to live their best love lives. She suggests surgical and non-surgical treatment options to improve female pelvic health. She helps to address symptoms of menopause, prolapse, pelvic pain syndromes, and other female sexual health issues. She is also an expert in Interstim and Botox therapy for bladder leakage.

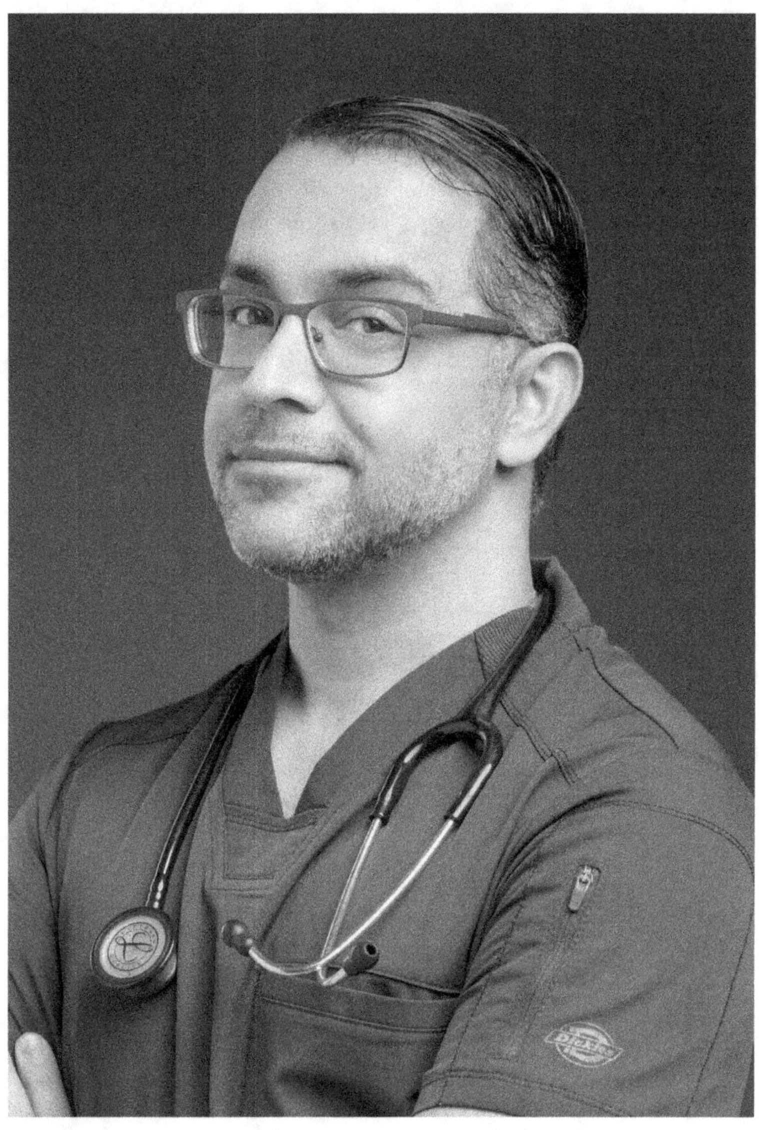

Dr. Siyamak Saleh

Dr. Siyamak Saleh

Dr. Siyamak Saleh is a sexual health influencer with more than three million followers on various social media sites. He is popularly known as the TikTok doctor and is the first from South Africa to be verified on the platform. His work in sexual and reproductive health advocacy is aimed at spreading awareness and driving positive change among people. Dr. Saleh studied medicine at the Lomonosov Moscow State University and later worked in cardiothoracic surgery research at the University of Cape Town. He educates young people about sex and helps older people overcome sexual dysfunction and improve sex. He busts popular myths around sex and speaks extensively about the sexual health of men and women.

ENDNOTES

SEXUAL HEALTH IS A PREDICTOR
OF OVERALL QUALITY OF LIFE
By Dr. Felice Gersh

References:

1. https://www.ncbi.nlm.nih.gov/pmc/articles/PMC6056803/
2. https://pubmed.ncbi.nlm.nih.gov/20822287/
3. https://www.unm.edu/~gfmiller/cycle_effects_on_tips.pdf
4. https://pubmed.ncbi.nlm.nih.gov/17688380/
5. https://www.ncbi.nlm.nih.gov/pmc/articles/PMC9218393/

MATCH.COM & OTHER DATING WEBSITES –
HOW THEY CHANGED OUR WORLD
By Navin Ramachandran

References:

1. https://www.ncbi.nlm.nih.gov/pmc/articles/PMC8646397/
   #spc312643-bib-0023
2. https://journals.sagepub.com/doi/full/10.1177/1069031X211073821
3. https://www.ncbi.nlm.nih.gov/pmc/articles/PMC2739403/

THE ART OF BEING DESIRELESS AT
THE HEIGHT OF DESIRE — WHAT THIS
MEANS AND WHY IT'S IMPORTANT
By Margot Anand

References:

1. https://www.ncbi.nlm.nih.gov/pmc/articles/PMC5641453/

WHY WE NEED SEX EDUCATION FOR ADULTS
By Dr. Kelly Casperson

References:

1. https://www.researchgate.net/publication/227680823_Association of_Lubricant_Use_with_Women's_Sexual_Pleasure_Sexual_ Satisfaction_and_Genital_Symptoms_A_Prospective_Daily_Diary_Study

2. https://www.besthealthmag.ca/article/how-viagra-can-hurt- your-relationship/

HELPING BUST SOME SEX MYTHS & IMPROVE RELATIONSHIPS
By Siyamak Saleh

References:

1. https://www.thelancet.com/journals/lancet/article/ PIIS0140-6736(15)61449-0/fulltext

2. https://www.ncbi.nlm.nih.gov/pmc/articles/PMC4558040/

3. https://www.ncbi.nlm.nih.gov/pmc/articles/PMC3731873/

4. https://www.eurekalert.org/news-releases/488474

5. https://www.healthyagingpoll.org/sites/default/files/2018-05/ NPHA-Sexual-Health-Report_050118_final.pdf